Beauty & Skin

— Reflections in Health Care —
Practical Approach to Look Younger

Hugo Romeu, M.D.

Beauty & Skin

Reflections in Health Care
"A Practical Approach to Look Younger"

Hugo Romeu, M.D.

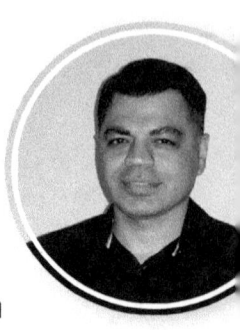

Revision & Editing by Amit Suneja

Amit Suneja is a serial entrepreneur, who has started, bought, built, and sold businesses related to natural health alternatives and skin care.

Amit is a graduate of 'The College of William and Mary;" best known as the alma mater of George Washington and Thomas Jefferson. Like many of the alumni , Amit is a prolific writer, provocateur and thinks outside of the box. Though he comes from successful Wall Street ventures, and has a proven track record in marketing; A near death experience was the catalyst that triggered Amit to Relentlessly pursue the discovery of natural health alternatives.

Although he does not have an educational background in Health Sciences , today many prominent physicians seek Amit's consultation regarding natural health alternatives; because of his formulations, and proven track record in developing products for the health and beauty industry.

Amit has created companies from the ground up which have rendered millions of dollars in revenue, and more important has assisted thousands in recovering their health.

He currently is involved in a score of innovations in the beauty industry, vitamins and supplements, as well as stem cell research and applications.

Contents
Introduction

Introduction

One day I asked a friend, a published author, Carlos Berenguer; to assist me in copywriting several topics related to Skin Care, Research, and health in general. The impetus was the realization that several of my works were being used in web sites by companies not authorized to do so.

Over a one month period Carlos showed me several hundred pages of work, which varied from philosophy to histology and research medicine. The topics are random at best, not initially intended for a book. After taking a look at the compiled body of work, it became obvious that perhaps there were three separate books: One focused on science and physical health, one on pharmaceutical research and treatment of common ailments, and one on the spiritual foundation of life dedicated to the practice of Medicine.

This is the first of the three. We will show an array of articles prepared for one of several ventures in the last two years. My professional background is in Medicine, Pathology, Education and Research.

The most important lesson here is a belief that life has meaning, and how you live has consequences.

This is a meager attempt to share a personal vision, which is common ground for every concerned doctor, student or patient. This book has more significance if it is interactive. Please forward your comments, ideas and perspectives to Hugo@ Romeuclinical.com or dr.hugoromeu@yahoo.com

Acknowledgements

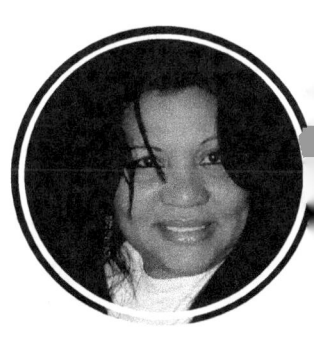

My life would have no meaning or significance without my family. It would be an empty mish mash of random thought and behavior. Instead everything I think and do has communal consequences.

If there is success, the ones I love, support and share with me. If there are pain and failure, they are by my side to give me strength and hope.

That being said, my wife Francis Zulueta Romeu, who has been my side for over 30 years, deserves the first mention. Without her constant reminder of how important it is to be honest and ethical, and her unwavering support, my life would be meaningless.

I would not exist if were not for my Mother and Father, Enna and Eduardo Romeu.

They showed me the importance of family and work ethic. Through them I clearly saw that anything was possible with hard work and persistence.

Srila Prabhupada introduced me to Vaisnavism and Vedic philosophy.

Since my teen years to the present, the chanting of the maha mantra, and devotional service solidify and give meaning to this blessed existence.

Hugo Romeu, MD

○────────────────────────────────○

om ajnana-timirandhasya jnananjana-salakaya
caksur unmilitam yena tasmai sri-gurave namah

I was born in the darkest ignorance, and my spiritual master opened my eyes with the torch of knowledge. I offer my respectful obeisances unto him.

○────────────────────────────────○

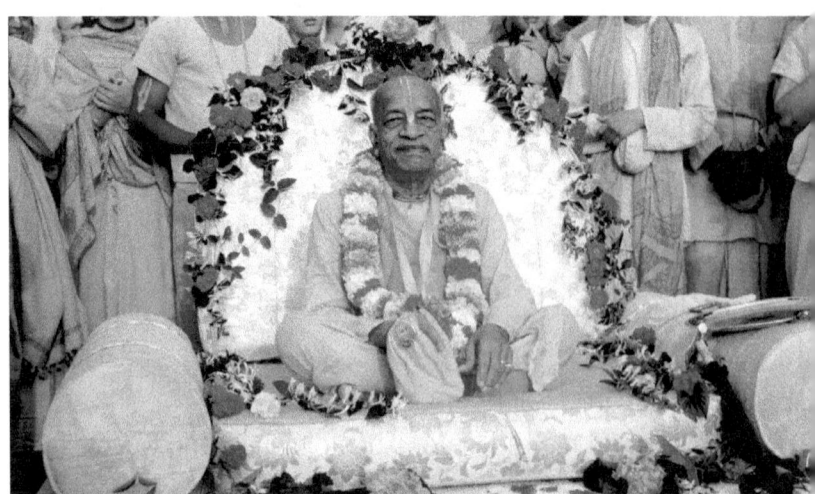

Chapter One
The big lie: Beauty is Only Skin Deep

The clock is ticking and calendar months progressing faster than before.

The older you get... the more time tends to fly faster, doesn't it?

No matter how pure your diet, or degree of tranquility achieved, the wear and tear that comes along with aging will manifest... sooner or later. Every organ begins to change loosing elasticity. Signs of diminished organ functional capacity become evident.

We must accept the changes as the natural course, but you don't have to sit back and watch the show unfold.

Before I discuss the ways to minimize, delay, conceal and at times cure the effects of aging on the skin, you should have a basic understanding of the terms and description of each complication. This way the method of treatment is an informed personal choice.

¡Make the rigth choices!

Chapter Two
Genetic constitution

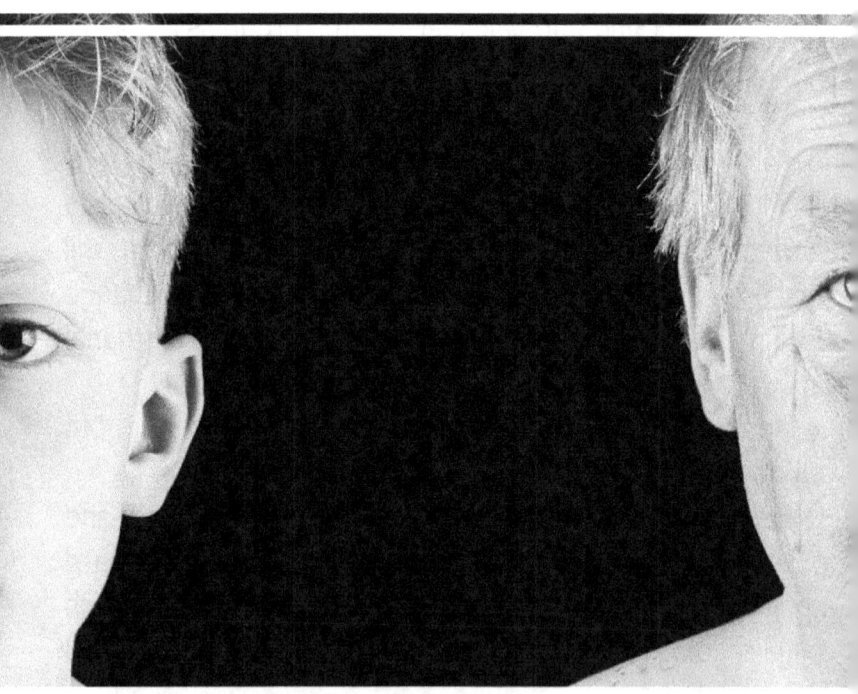

There are certain things that just "are", like your genetic constitution. Your genes are yours forever, no altering them. Depending on your genetic constitution, at times you are at the mercy of your genetics and at times you can alter the "appearance" of your genetics to look beautiful and attractive.

For example, were you aware that the distance between your eyes determines how beautiful you look?

Yes, if there are less than 12 centimeters separating each eye the eyes appear too close together.

There is not much you can do if you have less than 12 centimeters between your eyes.

However, if you do, you would look better wearing glasses. Also, prominent cheekbones make one look beautiful and this characteristic is impossible to alter. Other characteristics such as sagging jowls and a droopy neck, or perhaps a small chin: can be improved with surgical techniques.

Thick, Angelina Jolie like lips look luscious and inviting, that is plain and simple. If for some reason you have thin lips, they can be corrected with skin filler injections.

There are cultural differences, but there are common denominators shared by any genetic or opinionated imprints.

In some countries thin skinny woman are seen as ugly, whereas obese woman are found attractive.

There are regions where body tattoos and piercings are attractive, while in another regions they are repulsive. A full head of hair, long neck, big eyes, wide shoulders, tall stature are all common trans-cultural denominators.

Shiny, glowing skin is a universal attraction and rates as the #1 characteristic that determines beauty.

Lucky for you — shiny glowing skin can be had even if you weren't born with it.

The semblance of health is no different than the reflection of happiness: one just appears to glow.

This glow is a twofold manifestation. It is the evidence of healthy diet and positive attitude, and it is also how you want your skin to be perceived.

There are two forms of images to consider.

One is what others see and the other is how you see of yourself.

Both are important. Our interest is to focus on an objective scenario, you; consider how to improve the landscape. In the interim we must utilize the human hard drive, to process all the data.

By this I mean take into consideration everything you know and are learning about the skin, its structure and how it is altered by time, the environment and our habits, then look into the available tools, at your disposal, like this book, creams, exercise; and take a stance. Make the best of your constitution and age.

The destruction of beauty and the fight back.

Once the process of aging begins to show its true colors, the result is deterioration of the microscopic elements in the dermis, the collagen and elastin, with gradual thinning of the outer layer of skin, the epidermis.

Think of the way termites slowly destroy a nice house. At first there is no sign of these tiny creatures eating away at the wood, which keeps our home solid.

They move into the ceiling beams, walls, closets, and are persistently, hacking away at whatever is around. For so long only an expert can notice their presence. Eventually the damage is visible to the naked eye.

However, don't panic.

The good news is, even at late stages there are solutions.

The only difference is that the action needed to restore the original appearance needs to be more drastic.

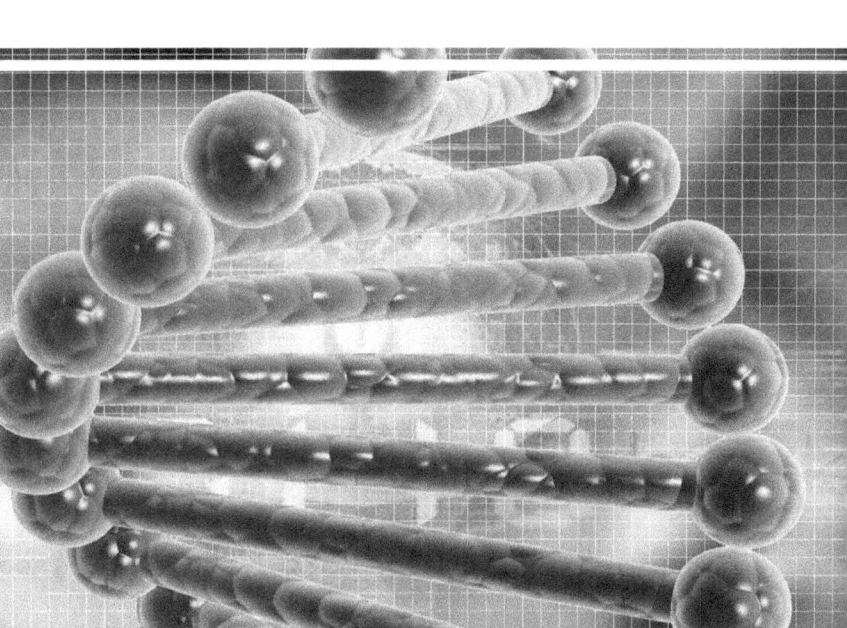

In the face we are looking for that natural glow, the expression of health and vigor. The glow even if it is lost can be recaptured.

It is never too late to make changes in your daily routine that can have a long term benefit. By using the right skin creams, changing your diet, and taking care of exposure to the sun, wind and cold, you can gain back the shine that has been lost.

One of the most blatant lies is "beauty is only skin deep." A close second is "beauty is in the eyes of the beholder." Remember, your skin is the ambassador of your body, mind and spirit. Everything that goes on in your body and mind – is reflected in how your skin looks and feels.

A diplomat represents a country to the rest of the world, and your skin is what people see of you, hence it is the ambassador which represents your complex multifaceted make up.

For example, a common term to describe pre mature facial wrinkles is 'worry line'. It's true, if you are constantly worried, depressed or anxious; the constant facial expressions which reflect this inner feeling are permanently embedded on the skin surface.

Most chronic forms of disease have an external sign observe d during a routine physical exam. For example, chronic hepatitis, or obstruction of bile ducts cause bile to flow into the subcutaneous tissue; this is called icterus, or jaundice.

Beauty is always a two way street. Inner spiritual and organic health is represented by a shiny and firm skin tone. For the best cumulative result and optimal effect you have to do a bit more than just use a new cream.

Think of any discipline or goal desired. To achieve this goal there are usually many ways. In the case of beautiful shiny skin, we have to work on many fronts. Yes, it is essential to begin a reparative process by using skin creams that will provide both cosmetic and regenerative make over; but if your desire is the maximum change for the better, then you must work on your inner beauty and daily habits.

What do you see in the mirror? Is it your soul or liver? Can you see the vitamins flowing through the blood and into each cell? If you can make sure you don't step on your cape as you fly out the window Superman or Wonder Woman.

You see only the outer surface, the skin, hair, eyes, and lips. You cannot see all of the organs in your body, or the biochemical components flowing through all systems.

Be sure that everything living is bidirectional. If your skin is glowing, it makes you feel better. So the energy is bidirectional.

Pretty on the inside, see it on the outside. Reflect on the people you have met during your life which impressed you. Think of why. Where they successful, intelligent, good?

Now think of those which you remember because they seem just happy. I guarantee they all have some things in common.

One is that you can see the evidence of their inner accomplishments. Happy, successful individuals simply look better than those that are miserable; this is a fact of life. Thus this energy is bidirectional. Feel it on the inside, see it on the outside. If you can't see it, maybe there is a reparative process that will have to do at first. Let's address the changes, which are most common, in fact they are inevitable manifestations of a ticking clock.

Chapter Three
Skin Structure

Structure of the Epidermis

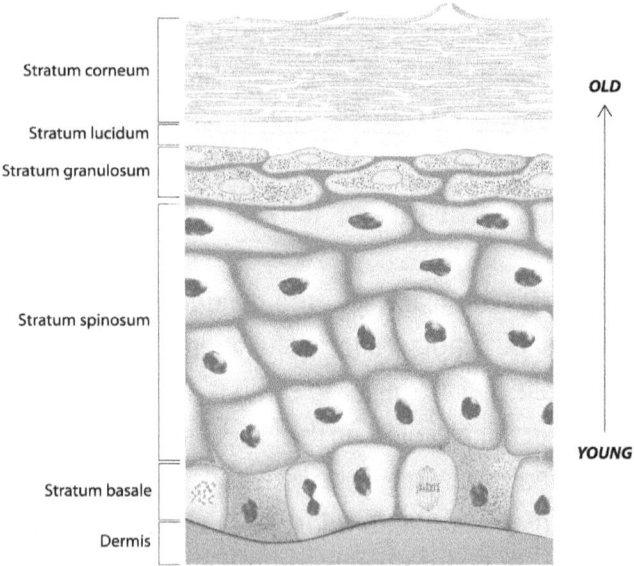

Stratum corneum

OLD

Stratum lucidum

Stratum granulosum

Stratum spinosum

YOUNG

Stratum basale

Dermis

Just after the skin cell is born it begins to produce a protein called keratin. The keratin is stored inside the cell. As the cell ages the keratin occupies more space within the cell and in the end is the only component left on the surface.

This layering of keratin actually becomes the outer protective barrier. Depending on the part of the body, the amount and thickness of this protective coat varies. Thickness is directly proportional to the protection needed.

The areas which are most sensitive have the thin keratin layer. In essence, keratin is the product of a dead skin cell. The gradual falling off is called exfoliation.

So the cells are born deep in the epithelium, grow, divide and die. Birth, growth, maturity and death: exactly like the cycles of our life, the epidermis follows the same progression. It is this same layer which must be permeated by the right concentrations of skin products to achieve success. The target site to prevent an accelerated decay is not the epidermis, but the dermis. So the area which is injected with Botox, or fillers, is the same area you want to alter with creams to address the aging process.

The dermis is the busy portion of skin. Hair follicles, nerve fibers, blood vessels, glands are held together by the glue of life; fibro connective tissue. On the most superior part of the dermis the ultraviolet rays of the sun stimulate the synthesis of Vitamin D. Energy is stored in fat deposits for later use, and the sense of pressure brings pleasure or pain, depending on the electric communication from the skin to the brain.

The glands are always busy regulating temperature and performing metabolic functions. Fibroblasts are all over the dermis, and it is these cells which produce collagen.

The loss of collagen means loose skin. Just as a loose bed spread forms a crease, loss of collagen means less elasticity and the appearance of wrinkles on the surface. There are a score of substances which can restore the natural smoothness and actually tighten the skin without that frighten look that Botox and plastic surgery can produce. In later chapters we will discuss the active ingredients of creams that really work by re hydrating and bringing a new found strength to the dermis.

The essential goal to prevent the formation of wrinkles is to hault the loss of collagen and the byproducts of elastin and hyaluronic acid. The immediate tendency is to force feed these ingredients back into the dermis. But it isn't that simple. If we look at the ultra-structure of the skin, the size of our pores will determine which ingredients pass beyond the protective keratin surface.

Life comes from life, and each cell is a reflection of the entire life experience. It is so amazing to see how cellular reactions mimic interpersonal experiences. Sounds a little far out, but consider this example.

Imagine a father with two sons. The father is trying to figure out how best to leave his children prepared to live without him. He just is not sure how. One day he decides to approach each differently and see which one is more successful.

To one son he gives a mass fortune, and says, "here my son, do with this gold as you wish." To the other he gives personal instruction on how to deal with obstacles, how to guide workers and simply pores all of his knowledge into him. To this son he does not give any money.

Well everyone knows that it's not just all about money. The way of continuity, stability and longer happiness is achieved by studying your surroundings and making the best of them. Sometimes the obvious is not so certain.

In the case of the skin, after a careful study of structure and function we can come to a few solid conclusions. Quickly we can come to the conclusion of what is missing. It's a bit harder to figure out how to replace it.

Chapter Four
Understanding Aging Skin

Let's say I had a magic wand and you could ask me one question — the answer to which would make you look years younger than your biological age... I'm guessing you'd ask, "Dr. Romeu what is the reason for my baby-smooth skin transforming into the crepe and crinkles of middle age... and how do I look years younger than my real age?"

Some of the answers lie in the nature of the skin itself. Just as anyone that drives a car does not need to be a mechanic,

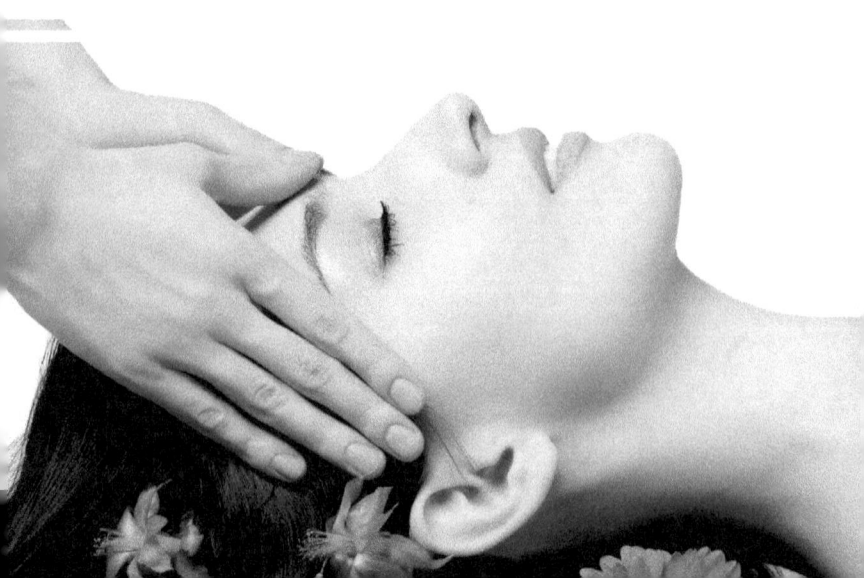

yet it is a good idea to know how to check the oil and change a flat tire. So also, it is a good idea for each one of us to learn the fundamentals about what makes up the skin and what it does.

Every bookstore, library and medical journal can be a source of detailed information. But you don't really need to know 90% of that information if you want to look young, and live a healthy life. Therefore, I will only tell you what you really need to know nothing more. You see, the most complex and mysterious structures were not created by man; they just exist from time immemorial. Science is the development of a detailed method to understand the forces of nature.

The human body is the perfect example of the harmonious relationship of so many different variables. The constantly changing human form is never static. From the moment of conception, cells quickly form, and develop into organs. These organs are all connected and interrelated in position, structure and function.

Anyone who studies a health related field must come to understand human anatomy to a varying level of complexity depending on the depth of studies. Whatever our profession, at some point we learn about the organ systems of the body. Compared to the brain, heart or lungs; the skin apparently is thought to be much easier to understand.

This is not the case. In fact we can say that the skin is a multi-tasking organ system. There are several different isolated functions of the skin.

Defense:

The first duty of the skin is to serve as a protective barrier. Your skin is the outer shield, which protects you from the elements and maintains the peace within. Like a busy factory in a windy city, the skin becomes the cement walls that keep the workers safe and the production constant. The skin is the barrier to all external physical, biologic and chemical invaders like the sun, detergents, pollutants, etc... In fact, it is the perfect protective barrier, because not only is it the first line of defense; the skin as a semi permeable membrane also makes sure that everything we need to maintain a healthy skin stays within the body. The idea is to keep the natural oils, fatty acids and moisture from escaping onto the surface. So the protection is twofold, by keeping harm way out, and important substances like hyaluronic acid in by not letting them be exposed directly to the atmosphere. This is the semi permeable function of the porous nature of the intercellular junctions.

Garbage Disposal:

The second task for the outer shield is similar to that of the kidneys, but on the surface of the body. We eliminate much of our body waste not only through urine and stool, but also through the glandular secretions realized in the dermis, in the form of micro glandular secretions. The natural oils of the skin or the lubricants needed to provide added protection as well as nutrition for the cell make up of the skin are also the products of these dermal secretions. The skin structures are able to eliminate waste while utilizing every single viable byproduct of routine metabolism. Keep in mind the skin creams we choose must blend with, replenish and exacerbate the function of the dermal secretions.

Temperature Regulator:

Yet another function of the skin is to act as a radiator, evaporator and insulator, keeping the bad out and the good in. As the internal or external temperature fluctuates, the skin roles with the punches. If there is a need to eliminate heat, the sweating process is kicked off. Just as the radiator in the car circulates the hydrants to cool the engine, the skin is the terminal route of circulating body fluids. As the body temperature rises water is excreted through the sweat glands, and the fluid lost is replenished from the intracellular fluids to the extracellular spaces. As the internal fluid levels get low, the thirst mechanism is triggered, and thus our desire to drink fluids and replenish them.

Sensual Stimulation:

The skin is the mediator of sensual stimulation. The sense of pressure brings pleasure or pain, depending on the electric communication from the skin to the brain. The peripheral nervous system actually ends in the nervous terminals located in the skin. The level of communication is extensive and complex between the environment and the brain. Everything we feel is the result of a complex electronic like exchange between our medium, the tiny nerve terminals in the skin; and the information, which is relayed to the brain via the nervous system. Everything from the cold wind, a foreign object or perhaps a gentle pat is translated into a sensation of pleasure or pain. So we can say that the skin is a complex information recovery system.

Understanding The Skin

It is essential to visualize the makeup of each portion to understand the effects of aging, and the ways to combat the downward spiral of accelerated decomposition of cells and more importantly, the "stuff" between cells, collagen and elastic fibers. You'll see the light in this knowledge in a few minutes.

The surface area of the skin makes up almost 20% of our entire body. Where the skin ends, the digestive, respiratory and urogenital systems begin.

Epidermis:

The epidermis is the top or outer layer of the skin. It is what we see with the naked eye. This outer surface is made up of 5 layers. These are actually 5 generations of skin cells, and you need a microscope to see them. At the junction between the dermis and the epidermis lies the basal or deep epithelial skin layer. These are the newborn cells as evidenced by the large nucleus and prominent genetic content within the boundaries of the nuclear membrane.

Skin cells are born in the dermal epidermal junction, and as they mature they rise like hot air into the outer and more

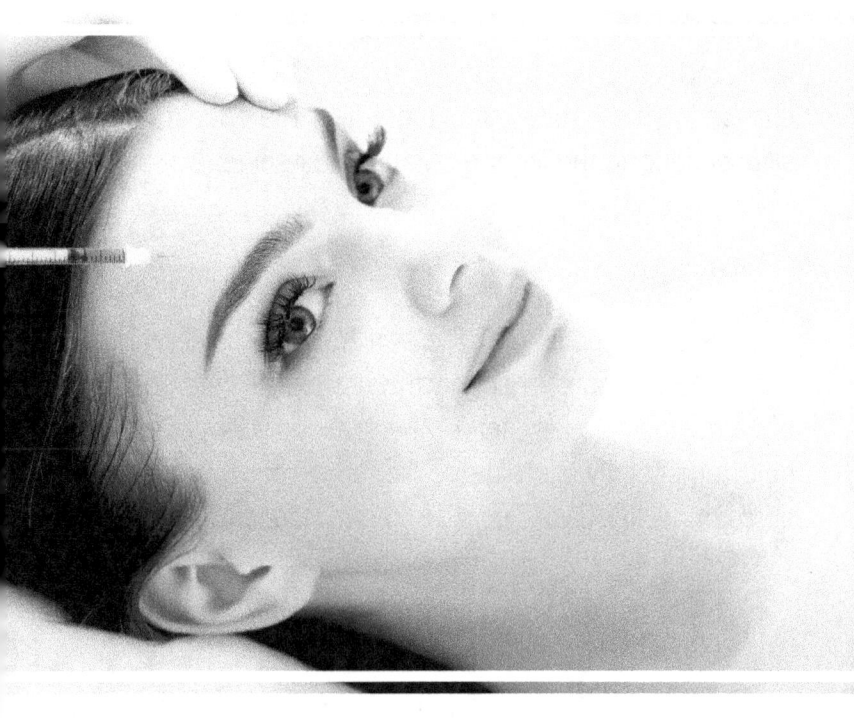

superficial layers. As the cells mature the nucleus becomes smaller and keratin begins to gradually abound in the cytoplasm of the cell. These cells are constantly being born, aging and dying. The skin epithelial cell has a life span of about 30 days. They are born at the base, and grow outwards until the dead cell looses all of its inner life components and settles on the surface. Just as a snake sheds and changes skin, so do we - only little by little, and in slow motion. The epithelium is what we see when glancing at someone. Thus your inner health and beauty become as evident as the viability of the outer shield. The concept of cellular turnover as described above is important to understand if you want to understand how the use of certain creams increases cellular turnover… thereby increasing the likelihood of looking younger. In addition I'll cover how the change in your habits can actually alter the appearance of the skin, enhancing the inner glow and outer shine.

Dermis:

The middle portion of the skin is called the dermis. This is the zone composed of connective tissues. It is the busy portion of skin. Hair follicles, nerve fibers, blood vessels, glands are held together by the glue of life; fibro connective tissue. The fibro connective tissue is made up of collagen and elastin fibers.

Collagen:

Collagen is an integral part of the skin's fabric and gives our skin its strength and elasticity. It is the main component of connective tissue, and is the most abundant protein in humans, making up about 25% to 35% of the whole-body protein content. Collagen, in the form of elongated fibril (like thread in a fabric), is mostly found in fibrous tissues such as tendon, ligament and skin, and is also abundant in cornea, cartilage, bone, blood vessels, the gut, and intervertebral disc.

The loss of collagen means loose skin. Just as a loose bed spread forms a crease, loss of collagen means less elasticity and the appearance of wrinkles on the surface.

There are a score of substances, which can restore the natural smoothness and actually tighten the skin without that "frightful look" that Botox and plastic surgery can produce. In later chapters we will discuss the active ingredients of creams that really work by re-hydrating and bringing a new found strength to the dermis.

Elastin:

Is a slinky like structure. It is a protein in connective tissue that allows many tissues in the body to resume their shape after stretching or contracting.

Elastin helps skin to return to its original position when it is poked or pinched.

Elastin is also an important load-bearing tissue in the bodies of mammals and used in places where mechanical energy is required to be stored.

The deeper portion of the dermis are composed of thicker fibers and laden with blood vessels, nerves and glands.

Fibroblasts:

The predominant cell in the dermis is the fibroblast. These cells are like the factory workers that produce collagen. There is a well know scientific term for this structural support component of the skin: the extracellular matrix. The collagen, elastin and fibrous elements swim within a gelatinous substance called hyaluronic acid.

The importance of hyaluronic acid cannot be overstated. Imagine an ocean of nutrition like amniotic fluid; this is the liquid that we live in during our gestational period in the womb. Well hyaluronic acid is a unique carbohydrate gel which is an essential component to facilitate moisturizing every viable structural component of the body; from the tendons and joints, eyes, brain to every single hair follicle. When choosing the perfect skin cream for you, make sure that the adequate amount and concentration of hyaluronic acid is present, or that you have found components that stimulate the natural production, for it is perhaps the single most important natural moisturizer.

Glands:

There are different glands in the dermis; the most important are sweat glands and sebaceous glands.

1. The sweat gland or apocrine and merocrine glands regulate our temperature by secreting fluid towards the surface.

2. The sebaceous gland secretes an oily product. The glands are always busy regulating temperature and performing metabolic functions.

Now you can understand how the multifaceted function and structure of the skin has specific purpose and function. Knowing this each individual can maximize the natural structure and functions of skin by taking the adequate measures to potentiate and assist your own god given defenses against the natural course of time.

Chapter Five
The secret to looking Young

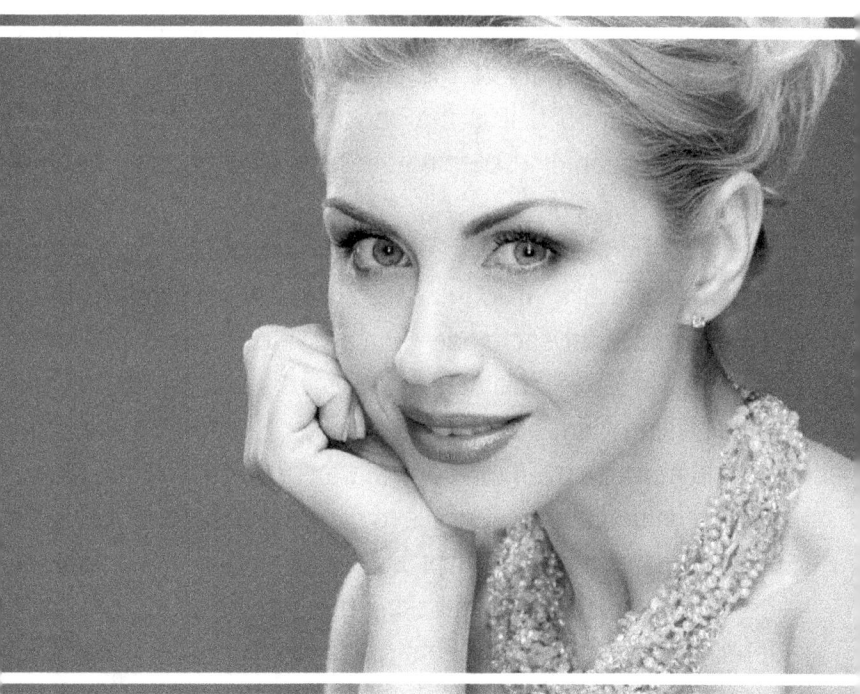

The essential goal to prevent the formation of wrinkles is to halt the loss of collagen and the by products of elastin and hyaluronic acid. If you look at the body as a mechanical structure, it will be simple to understand how a wrinkle is formed and what collagen, elastin and hyaluronic acid have to do with it. Every machine has similar components. Whether we are referring to a car, plane, lawn mower or human body. The engine, the electronic portion, the fuel system, exhaust, etc... depending on the sophistication of the design and complexity of the function the details of the structure are elaborated. No matter what the machine is, and what it does; it needs lubrication and shocks.

Well, in a nutshell the dermal matrix and its essential components are part of the sophisticated bodily lubrication and frame support. It is the shock absorber, the motor oil, the transmission fluid keeping the breathing machine flexible, strong and functional.

Hyaluronic acid has the unique capacity to attract and bind to water like no other structure. This carbohydrate or complex mucopolysacharide can carry more than 1000 times its weight in water. This natural polymer is not only the oil and transmission fluid, but also the shiny component of the paint job and perhaps even the applied wax to bring back the shine.

The immediate tendency is to force feed these ingredients back into the dermis. But it isn't that simple. If we look at the ultra-structure of the skin, the size of our pores will determine which ingredients pass beyond the protective keratin surface. (I'll talk about the importance of keratin and how it affects the skin in just a second.) For now, imagine your skin's outer layer as a giant siv, with pores of certain dimension. Only what is smaller than that pore will pass from one side to the next. There are different ways to penetrate the mechanical barrier.

1. You can force your way through by injecting fillers and nutrients past the porous barrier, as is the case with injectable fillers.

2. You can also combine the use of several agents like citric acid, retin, and coenzymes to stimulate the new production of hyaluronic acid within your skin. There are also absorbed molecular variants which will be absorbed and provide benefits. Substances that are the right size will go through the pore.

Keratin
Just after the skin cell is born it begins to produce a protein called keratin. Keratin is stored inside the cell. As the cell ages

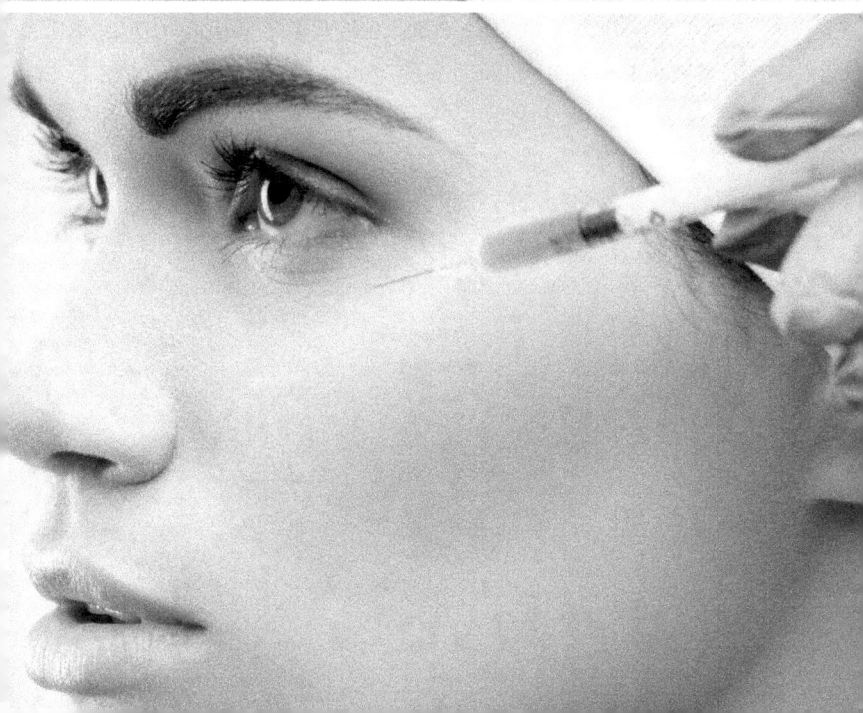

the keratin occupies more space within the cell and in the end is the only component left on the surface. This layering of keratin actually becomes the outer protective barrier. Depending on the part of the body, the amount and thickness of this protective coat varies. Thickness is directly proportional to the protection needed. The face, neck and arms all have a thick keratin layer; for they are in direct contact with the elements. The tips of the finger, and gentialia have very thin keratin layers, thus are the most sensitive. In essence, keratin is the REMNANT of a dead skin cell. The gradual falling off is called exfoliation. This is a fancy way of saying shedding old skin. Eliminating nonviable or dead unessential elements is the natural way to make way for the new and viable. By exfoliating the skin surface we can prepare to enrich and revitalize the skin so that the natural glow can be seen to its fullest.

Above is an actual cut of skin, which is stained to evaluate by the student or physician specialist.

Anatomy of the Epidermis

Dead cells flaking off at the skin surface

Stratum corneum
Stratum lucidum
Stratum granulosum

Stratum spinosum

Stratum basale
Dermis

Keratinocytes move up as they age

What Good Is All This Information?

The question to ask now is, "How is the above knowledge about the structure and function of the skin going to help me look younger?" Well, let's talk about the mighty wrinkle and see how the above information is so important to finding the cure.

The Mighty Wrinkle

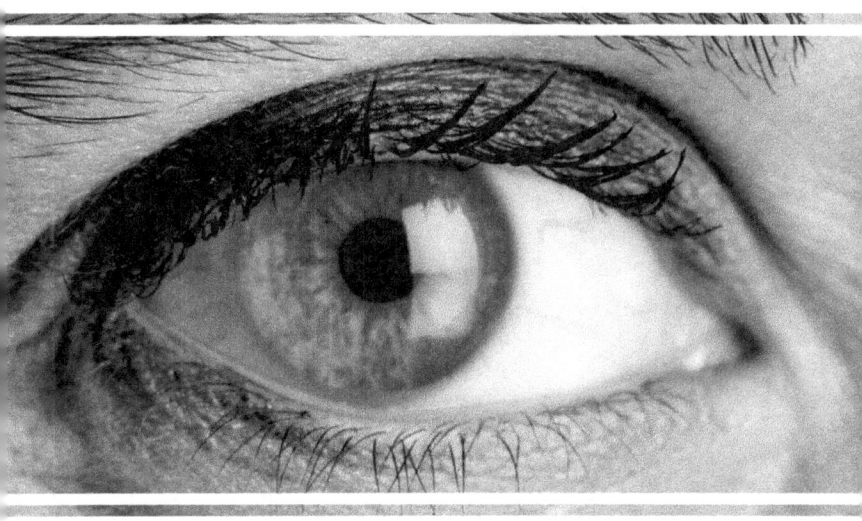

A wrinkle is a fold on the surface of our skin, apparently?
Wrong, a wrinkle happens in the dermis. The changes which lead to loss of collagen and elastin occur in the dermis. Aging is nothing more than putting miles, wear and tear, on your vehicle. As the calendar progresses so does the mileage. There are highway miles, and city miles. In other words every

machine has a proprietor who must maintain and upkeep for optimum appearance and function. As the structural elements in the dermis are utilized, whether consumed or just denatured, the skin becomes loose and the covering slips in between the cracks in the amour.

Sagging:

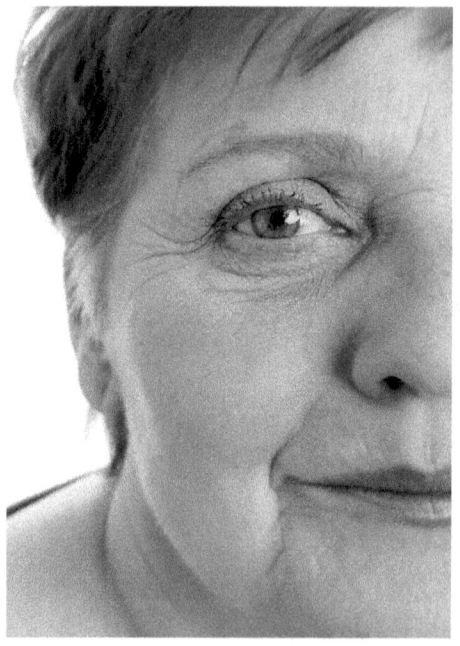

While the skin becomes loose there are other effects besides just wrinkles. Gravity will pull the weaker skin downwards causing sagging. Which is nothing more than the loss of tensual strength and elasticity of the skin?

Thinning Skin: The wear and tear brings on slower cell turnover in the epidermis, thus a thinner outer covering. Aging means thinner skin and being more sensitive to the outer and inner elements.

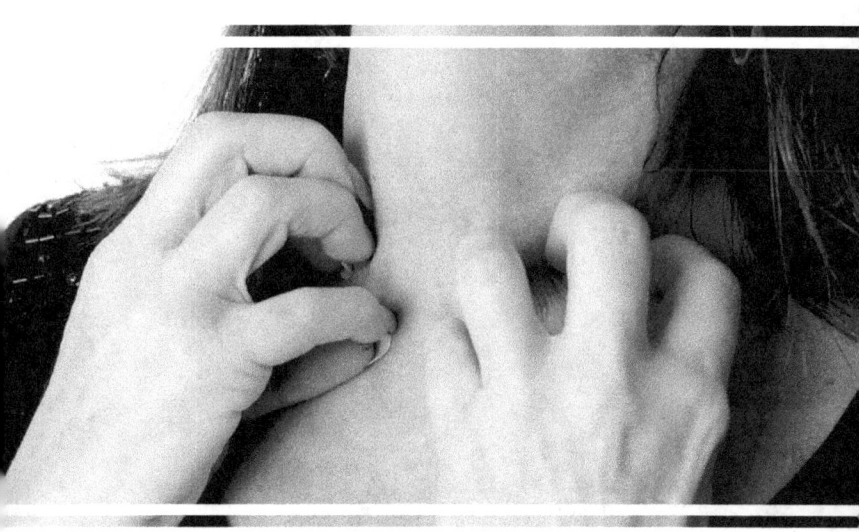

Hyperpigmentation: Remember the discussion of melanocytes and where they are situated in the epidermal structure. Well another phenomenon during aging is the uneven distribution, storage and elimination of melanin pigment. Thus the brown tincture begins to accumulate in undesired locations causing focal hyper-pigmentation or age spots.

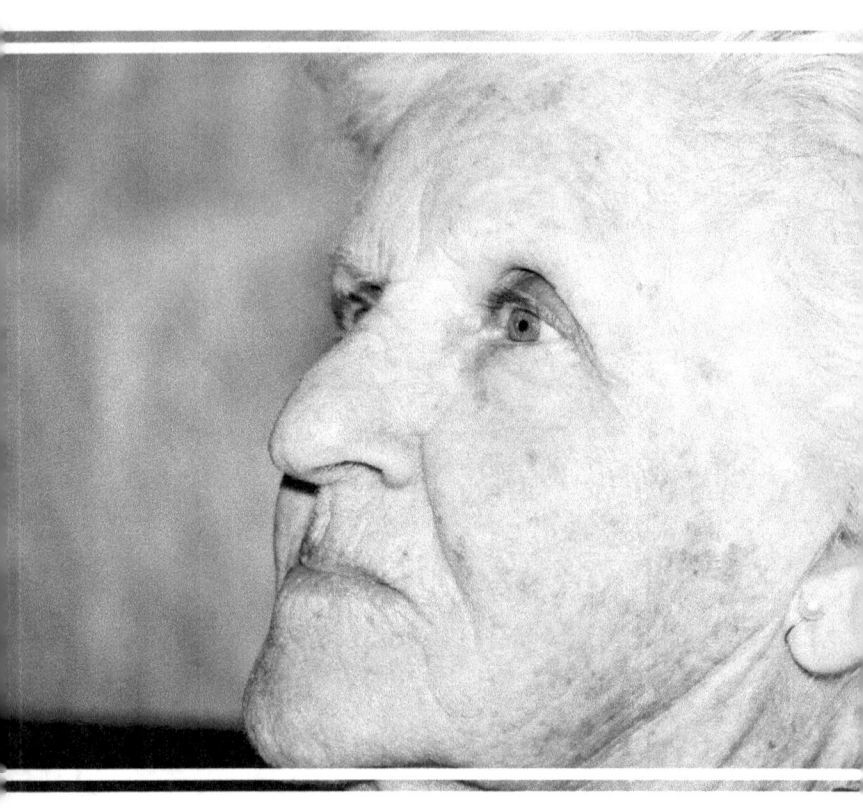

The Cure: By understanding each portion of the skin, we can begin to comprehend how to treat each worry. As I've already covered, the skin cells are born deep in the epithelium, grow, divide and die. Birth, growth, maturity and death: exactly like the cycles of our life, the epidermis follows the same progression. It is this same layer, which must be permeated by the right concentrations of skin products to achieve success.

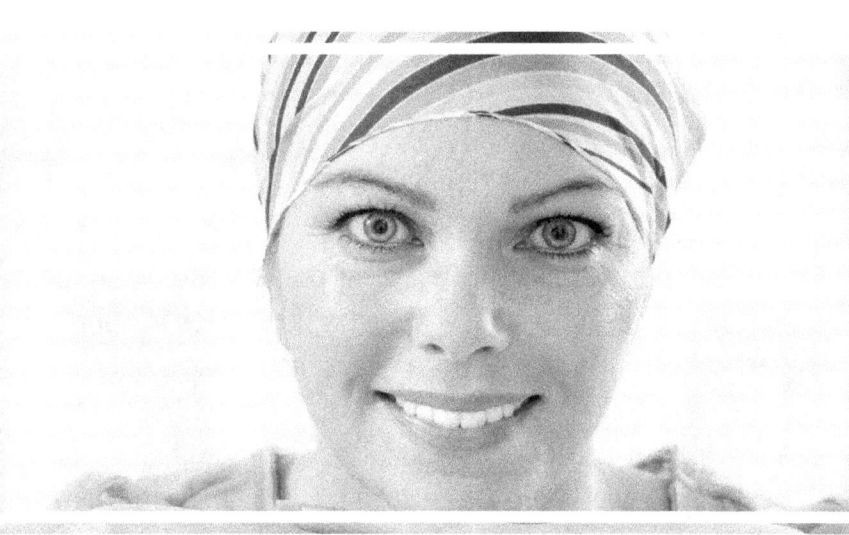

Remember, the target site to prevent an accelerated decay is not the epidermis, but the dermis. The area, which is injected with Botox, or fillers, is the same area you want to alter with creams to address the aging process. Cosmetic companies off course won't tell you this... they'll sell you products that "feel good" on the epidermis layer and all you have is a hope and a prayer to look young.

While we will touch on many of the common skin problems, as I've said before, the focus of this book is the ,'the wrinkle.' In the case of wrinkles, the point is to learn and teach how aging affects the skin, and then try assist individuals in looking younger than their physical age.

There are many options, including surgical or minimally invasive procedures, to yoga, to chanting meditation, to the application of creams, ointments and vitamins. Don't worry; I'll cover all the treatments available to you.

Let's Get Esoteric: Life comes from life, and each cell is a reflection of the entire life experience. It is so amazing to see how cellular reactions mimic interpersonal experiences. Sounds a little far out? Then consider this example.

Imagine a father with two sons. The father is trying to figure out how best to leave his children prepared to live without him. He just is not sure how. One day he decides to approach each differently and see which one is more successful.

To one son he gives a mass fortune, and says, "here my son, do with this gold as you wish." To the other he gives personal instruction on how to deal with obstacles, how to guide workers and simply pores all of his knowledge into him.

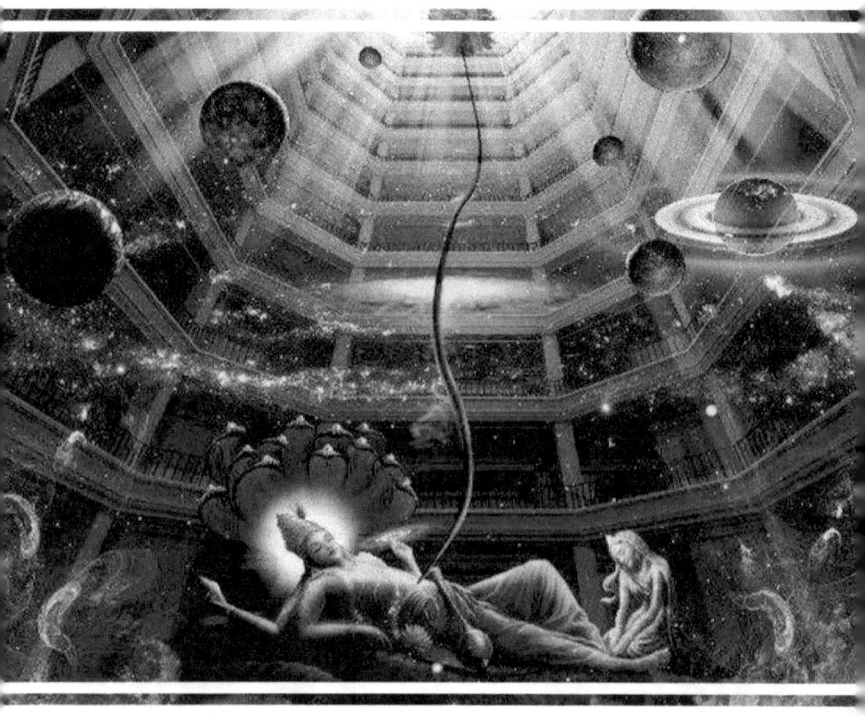

To this son he does not give any money.

Well everyone knows that it's not just all about money. The way of continuity, stability and longer happiness is achieved by studying your surroundings and making the best of them.

Sometimes the obvious is not so certain. In the case of the skin, after a careful study of structure and function we can come to a few solid conclusions.

1. Quickly we can come to the conclusion of what is missing.

2. It's a bit harder to figure out how to replace it.

3. By understanding this simplified explanation of the structure and function of the skin, you can begin to see how the proper mixture of ingredients and foods; from vitamins to mucopolysacharides can penetrate the outer barrier and stimulate the production of new collagen, elastin and hyaluronic acid in the dermis. This will cause a filling effect, much like a Botox injection, but in a natural and non-invasive fashion.

I'll cover the specifics of the "cure" in the next few chapters.

Chapter Six
The Wrinkle

Is there anyone on this planet that does not know what a wrinkle is? Well, if you don't, a wrinkle is a crease in the skin. There is a short and a long explanation of how this indented fold occurs, then develops. Let's try the middle of the road explanation. Have you ever noticed how a snare drum is constructed? There is a circular metal device, with a series of metal rods extending from the superior to inferior margins of the rim. On the surface, is a canvas made of leather or a synthetic simulation. All around the circular border of the overlying canvas there are connections which adapt the canvas to the rim by anastomosing the metal rods to the canvas border with an intermediary string like material. Using

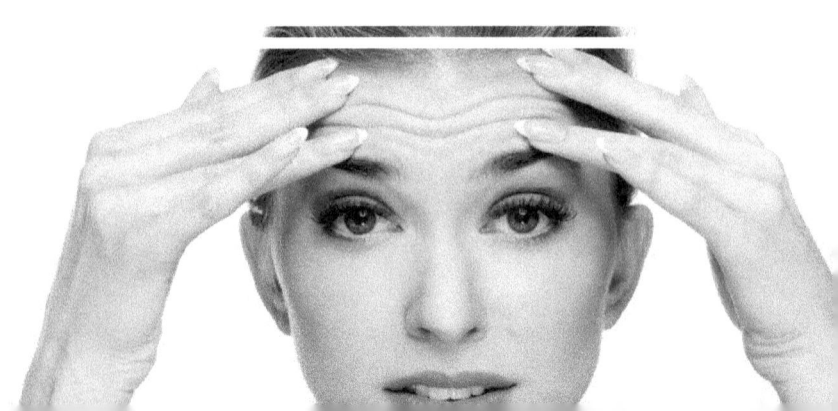

a special tool, the canvas is tightened until evenly stretched and tense.

The sound is now adjusted depending on the tightness of the overlying drum skin. If the skin is let loose, or a supporting structure breaks down, the drum skin is indented, creases are formed due to the looseness, and the sound is not good. OK. Now, try to refresh your basic histology lessons we have shared thus far. The collagen, elastin, fibroblasts and entire dermis are those supporting structures. Your skin is the overlying canvas pounded by the drumsticks. When there are problems due to the wear and tear effects of usage multiplied by time, the supporting structures of the skin break down, and the top caves in. Just like roof coming down when the beams are compromised, the skin folds inward when the dermis is compromised.

"Oh dreaded crease of time that no rhyming line can imitate.
This skin of mine with time has come to be what I hate.
Show me the way to fall in love again with that reflection.
The image in that mirror is my only connection.
With what people see of me."
You will never hear, "what a great thing
happened to me this morning.
I went to brush my teeth and noticed
the wrinkles on my face."
Not going to happen, ever.

Cigarettes smoking probably has the most negative effect on your skin. People who smoke have very distinctive wrinkles caused by the use of specific muscles and the high content of carbon monoxide in their blood.

Every time a smoker puffs on a cigarette, then blows the smoke out, they use muscles of the face to accomplish these tasks. The constant muscular contractions, then relaxations

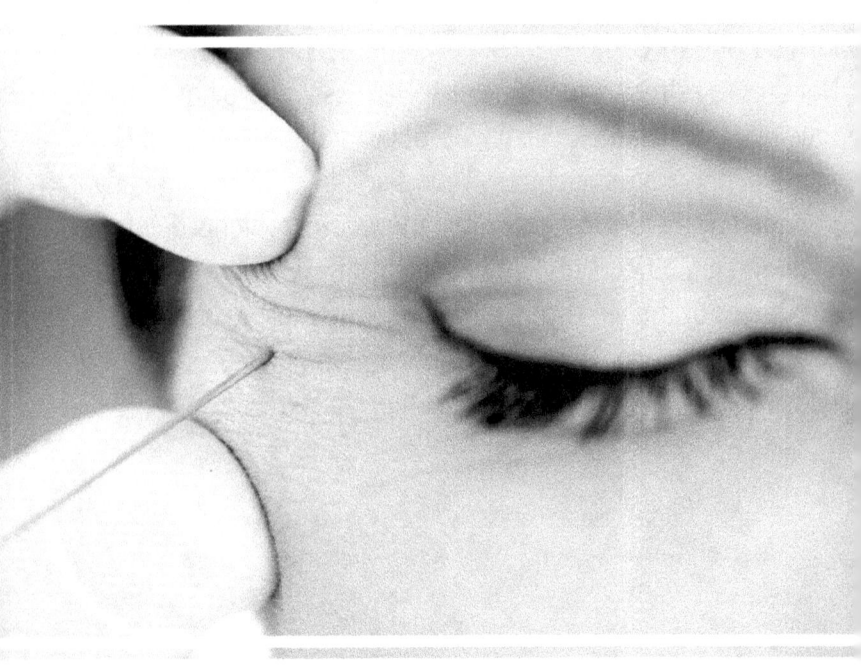

carry the overlying skin along for every ride. The results are distinctive deep wrinkles that tail away from the borders of the lips down and out, like the whiskers of a cat.

The sun is also a very corrosive agent causing severe damage to the skin.

It's too late to lament the hours spent laying out by the pool or beach with your reflector and bottle of baby oil. Time to get out of the sun and into the shade, the cool soothing place with the right attitude.

The first step is to objectively assess the damage. Sometimes it is best if an unbiased observer is with you for this. Remember the section about skin typing; it's time to put your new found knowledge to use. After determining how deep is your wrinkle, and how dry, try to map out a plan. For this you will need professional help. Anyone who is concerned about their wrinkles' deserves the opportunity to improve their appearance, by minimizing the appearance of the facial crevices. There are many types of professionals with expertise on skin care. Each phase and advancement of the aging process has different tools and experts to wheel them. The dermatologist, cosmetologist, plastic surgeon, cosmetics company, or maybe your Avon lady; any or all can join the team. We will discuss the role of each professional, and how you can decide which ones to take shelter of.

Back to square one. Can you answer this question? What causes a wrinkle?

Our plan must come with a way to replenish and or stimulate the proteins, vitamins and even cells that have been lost. The way is to protect and hydrate, relax and paralyze the fibers. Have you ever read about botulism poisoning? Well, the victim becomes paralyzed, unable to move or react to any stimulus. Botox is derived from the same venom, but used in a very small dose to cause a type of partial paralysis. The effect is to tighten the fibro muscular structures and stretch out the skin. If you can see the problem you can visualize the solution, and severity of wrinkle. No matter the age wrinkles can appear, and you have to take the time and take a stance. Beauty is only enhanced by the cure of wrinkles.

The effectiveness of creams will depend on the composition and active ingredients. The use of prescription creams and retinoid has been documented to improve wrinkles. The active ingredients are often the same but mixed in different proportions. Antioxidants, alpha hydroxyl acids, Co enzyme Q10 have shown great promise. An array of vendors pushing magic formulas, like snake oil vendors in the wild west, hide behind the loose restrictions that a cosmetic cream has over an FDA regulated prescription medication. The flip side of this coin is that many natural and non toxic compounds without the need to be regulated by drug enforcement agencies are the very stuff that creams can be made from. The shortcoming is that a lesser degree of active components are often found in non-prescription creams. We will discuss in detail our recommendations in a chapter to follow, along with alternative therapies with different levels of invasiveness.

The Outer Shield

A colleague of mine who is familiar with the work of my practice first laughed when I told him that I wanted to write about wrinkles. This is what 8 years of graduate and post graduate education, along with 31 years of experience led to. The way you see anything is altered by the depth of your perception. The familiar line, a little information is dangerous, is not as lethal as taking simple truth for granted. The purpose of my career is to better the lives of my patients. It is rare to actually save anyone's life, or radically alter the course of a disease, but it is possible to offer advice and alternatives

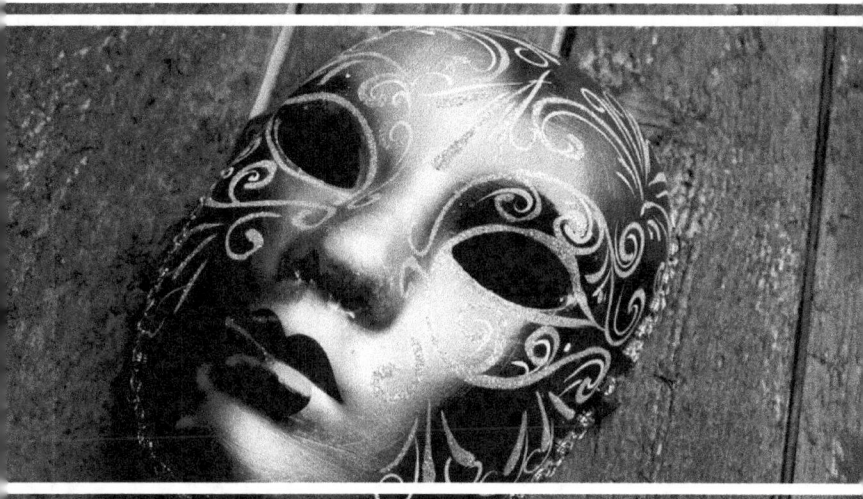

that can improve the quality of someone's life. The more time I reflect on the most common concerns of my patients, friends and family, the more I realize that it is the most obvious concerns stare us in the face.

Physicians, by vocation, are more than just health care providers. We are here to listen to all the concerns of our patients. They all come for a well fitness check, or a physical concern; but during their visit many topics are discussed. Some talk about their kids, husbands, friends or perhaps their job.

After 31 years of practicing medicine and multitasking in the arena, I have come to the conclusion that all of my patients have a few things in common, eventually.

As a young scientist, the hunger to understand complex issues seems to obscure simple realities. One of the first systems a medical student must learn is the Integumentary

System. This is a fancy way of saying the skin. The skin is in fact the largest organ of the body , it is our shield and filter from the outer world.

As a younger physician, dealing with vanity was never a priority. When ones patients grow older, and one follows in the same path, the way you look becomes a source of insecurity. Common knowledge shows us that new relationships, jobs and interpersonal experience is pendant on how one projects, and how you are visualized. In the end one word means so much to describe a common problem in self-perception, and first impressions, 'wrinkle'.

Have you ever lost something? Searched all over, only to find the object of your desire right before you?

Human anatomy is what we see at first glance. Histology is what we see using different types of microscopes. The accumulation of new knowledge about the cellular make up of our form leads to a complex vision of the human of the human body.

Just a few blocks from my home, is a street that bears the name of a journeyman, an adventurer dedicated to the pursuit of eternal youth? Ponce de Leon thought he found spring waters in Florida that led to eternal youth.

Over the years, facets of my practice have been dedicated to understanding cellular structure and function. In fact much of my time has been dedicated to consulting other physicians. As a surgical pathologist histology is the building block of how to understand function and change. Histology means the structure and appearance of cells, and their relation to each other. The first years of medical school are dedicated to learning about the normal body. The naked eye, the microscope, an x-ray…each offer a unique picture and puzzle piece to grasping the interrelationship of every body system.

So the book that follows is the attempt of a physician to deal with a very common and universal issue: we all age. That does not mean we have to take a passive stance and just allow the normal physiologic process to move forward at a rapid pace.

Somehow or another all roads lead to self-confidence. One reflects a self-image by the way one walks, talks and communicates.

The skin is what we see when glancing at a person. We don't see the heart, lungs or kidneys, but the skin. We should never underestimate the complexity and importance of the outer shield. The eyes are the window of the soul, and the skin is our protection, mediator of sense, and regulator of energy.

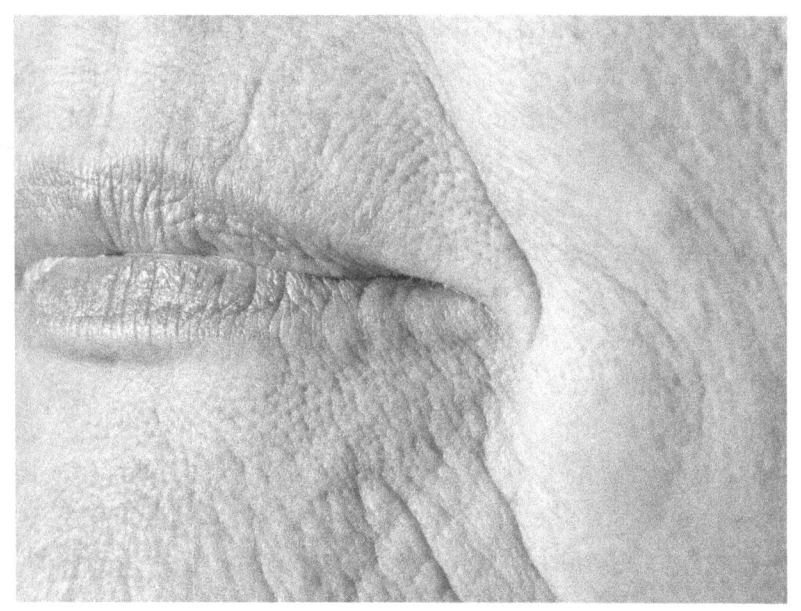

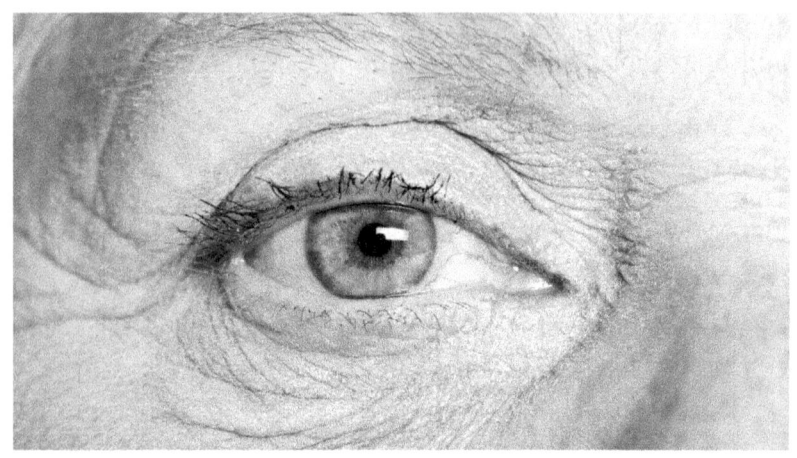

The way you look is the composite of so many factors. Independent of each factor are common variables to adjust the outer reflection, the shield, the skin.

Well, this is how I feel about writing this book. For so many years I have studied all of the details of the skin. Written reports about inflammatory diseases such as lupus or psoriasis. At other times, studied and discussed malignant lesions of the skin such as melanoma or squamous cell carcinomas. After thousands of patient interviews, and elaboration of just as many reports describing results, and treatment. The last thing I could imagine is that there would be an interest in writing about wrinkles. After all what does a wrinkle have to do with surgical pathology?

No matter who you are, where you're from or what you do; every morning we rise from sleep and make our way to the bath room. The light goes on; the water is adjusted to certain temperature by a turn of a knob, than we stare directly forward. And there it, the first daily glance at our face. As the years go by, new wrinkles begin to appear. To this date I have never met anyone that is happy with the site of a new wrinkle. Just as there are so many different body types and personalities to go with them, each has a different way to address a problem. Some are quite simple, and there are a wide array of gradients. My job as a physician is to ponder and study how to help my patients deal with their concerns. It's not just a common cold, or belly ache that I deal with daily. My concerns are no different than any of theirs. Not only are we all concerned about how we feel physically and emotionally, we all wonder if we look our best.

For the last several years there has been a tendency to explore alternative ways to assist patients. My practice has undergone extensive changes, call it an evolution.

Criteria about THE WRINKLE

Oh dreaded crease of time that no rhyming line can imitate.
This skin of mine with time has come to be what I hate.
Show me the way to fall in love again with that reflection.
The image in that mirror is my only connection.
With what people see of me.
You will never hear,
"what a great thing happened to me this morning.
I went to brush my teeth and noticed
the wrinkles on my face."
Not going to happen, ever.

The question is, do the wrinkles bother you? It's too late now to lament all the cigarettes smoked, or hours spent laying out by the pool or beach with your reflector and bottle of baby oil. Time to get out of the sun and into the shade, the cool soothing place with the right attitude. The first step is to objectively assess the damage. Sometimes it is best if an unbiased observer is with you for this. Remember the section about skin typing, it's time to put your new found knowledge to use. After determining how deep is your wrinkle is, and how dry, try to map out a plan. For this you will need professional help. Anyone who is concerned about their wrinkles deserves the opportunity to improve their appearance, by minimizing the appearance of the facial crevices. There are many types of professionals with expertise on skin care. Each phase and advancement of the aging process has different tools and experts to wheel them. The dermatologist, cosmetologist, plastic surgeon, cream entrepreneur; or maybe your avon lady; any or all can join the team.

Back to square one. Can you answer this question? What causes a wrinkle?

Take a look at the photos below. Notice the mesh of fibers that constitute the frame within the dermis. Our plan must come with a way to replenish and or stimulate the proteins, vitamins and even cells that have been lost. The way is to protect and hydrate, relax and paralyze the fibers. If you can see the problem you can visualize the solution. zone and severity of wrinkle advanced changes even the young grow old.

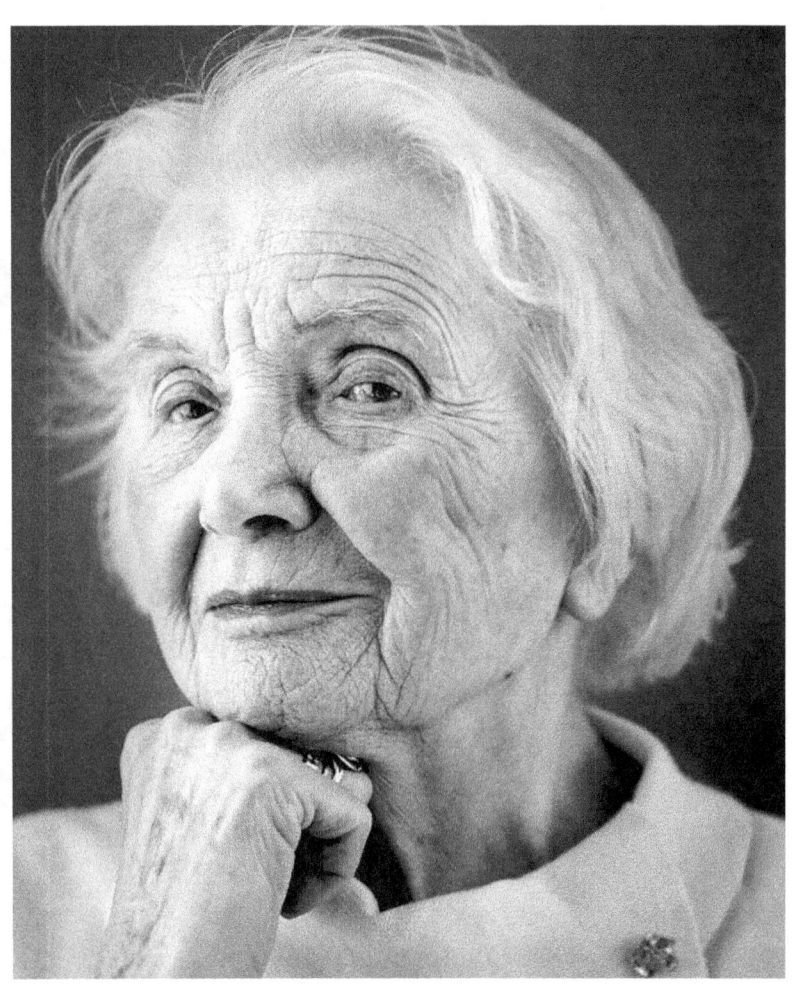

No matter the age wrinkles can appear, and you have to take the time and take a stance. Beauty is only enhanced by the cure of wrinkles.

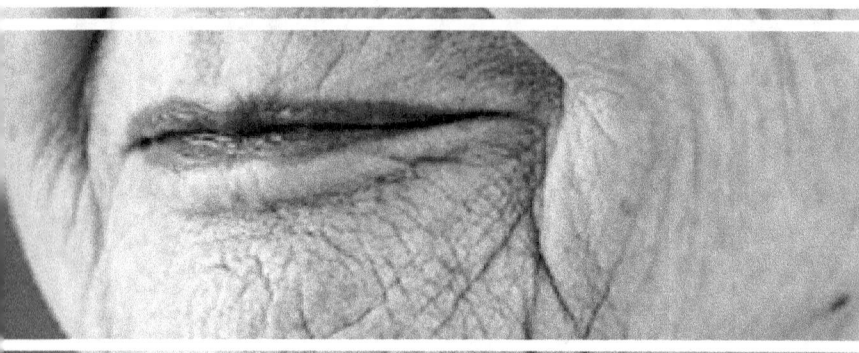

The effectiveness of creams will depend on the composition and active ingredients. The use of prescription creams and retinoid has been documented to improve wrinkles. The active ingredients are often the same but mixed in different proportions.

Antioxidants, alpha hydroxyl acids, Co enzyme Q10 have shown great promise.

An array of vendors pushing magic formulas, like snake

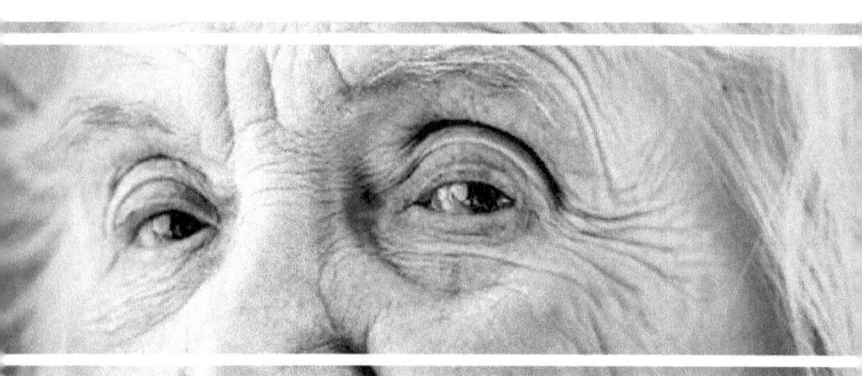

oil vendors in the wild west, hide behind the loose restrictions that a cosmetic cream has over an FDA regulated prescription medication. The flip side of this coin is that many natural and non-toxic compounds without the need to be regulated by drug enforcement agencies are the very stuff that cream scan be made from. The short coming is that a lesser degree of active components are often found in non-prescription creams. We will discuss in detail our recommendations in a chapter to follow, along with alternative therapies with different levels of invasiveness.

Chapter Seven
Dry Flaky Skin, Eczema

Just as dreaded as the wrinkle, but with a worse potential for escalating damage, is eczema. This is one of the most misunderstood and misquoted terms in medical literature. Unfortunately it has spilled over into the cosmetic industry.

Eczema is not only a tough word to spell it's a complex condition of the skin and part of the aging process. The area of skin with the thinnest protective layer, the epidermis, is the segment most vulnerable. There are experts in skin disease that believe the term eczema should not even be used anymore, because there is no consensus on the meaning. In medical libraries entire sections are filled with books about the effects of aging on the skin. It was surprising to discover how much information is just plain confusing. The term itself:

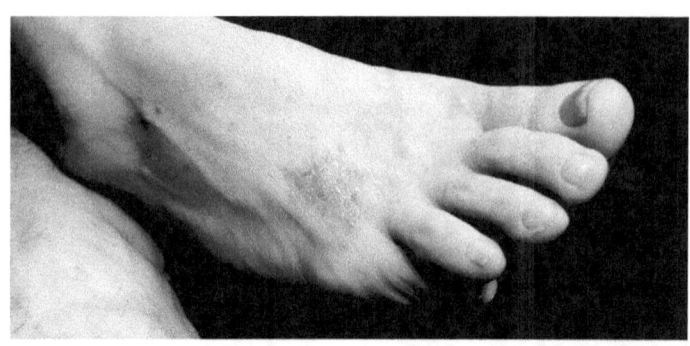

eczema, is used in many different ways depending on the background of the author. What most authors mean when they use the term eczema is atopic dermatitis.

Any word ending in 'itis' in a medical book means, there is inflammation there. For example dermatitis means inflammation of the skin. Arthritis means inflammation of the joints, and so forth. In Greek the word eczema means to boil out. In fact on a microscopic and later gross level, that is exactly what happens. As we age, the skin becomes thinner, and depending on your skin type and season there are little cracks in the armor. The great protector is now vulnerable to both external influences and manifestations of inner signals. Eczema happens where there is a weakness in the skin and the sign becomes the symptom. The difference between a sign and symptom — a sign is something that is visible and observed by a keen eye and a symptom is something that is manifested into a disease process. So for example, one of the first signs of eczema is dry skin. If this gets worse and develops into a persistently growing area of scaling skin; than a symptom evolves. Eczema is really an allergic reaction causing the formation of dry and itchy areas with varying degrees of severity. First you must be genetically predisposed, then the weather and everything around you triggers the reactions. Perhaps a pet, detergent, stress, diet or simple dust can cause a chain of reactions ending in a red patchy skin surface, that is ugly and itches. Sometimes in medicine those complaints that are passed over as not so serious, are the ones that bother the patients most.

In many societies the physician is looked up to as an individual that is very knowledgeable, wise beyond his years. This assumed wisdom is often just a misconception. Doctors are no different from anyone else, except they spent more time in school learning a trade; A job which is always changing by new discoveries, both in diagnostics and treatment.

The doctor doesn't always have the answers, but too often physicians rely on certain nebulous terms to categorize a disease or symptom.

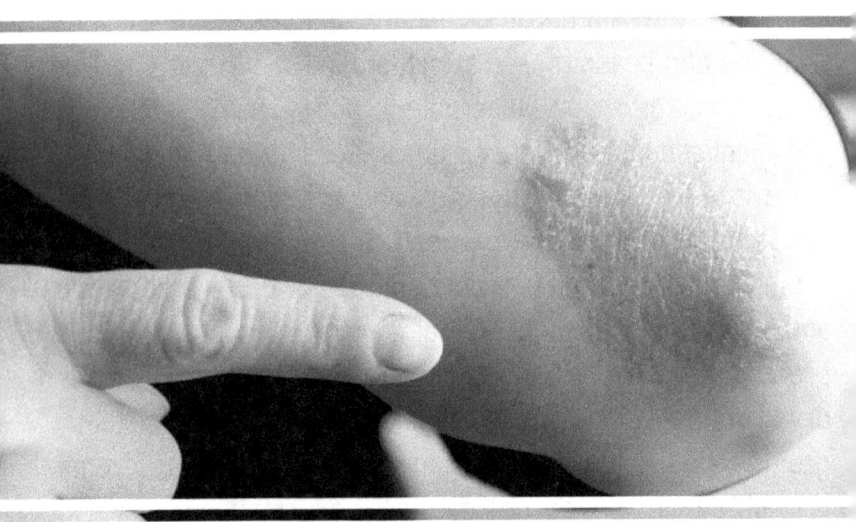

Eczema is one of those dumping ground terms. A rash, dry area, itchy spot, red patch...don't know what it is? Let's just call it "eczema", an esoteric sounding word which seems to accurately describe a legitimate affection of the skin.

As a health care provider a thorough history and physical examination of the concerned person is warranted. The underlying patterns and trigger stimuli that start the skin reaction.

There must be great care to analyze and find the appropriate personal care to minimize and prevent the occurrence of dry, flaky snake like skin. Always be ready for the winter and dry climates by applying natural remedies and avoiding irritants, especially soaps and detergents.

Keep your skin hydrated with aqueous creams and sheltered from the tempered environment. It is definitely not a good idea to daydream while taking a long hot shower, because the pores of your skin will open up and necessary natural oils will ooze out through the wide open spaces.

The subsequent effect will be a drier depleted skin.

Try to use warm water and just cleanse your body with a healthy cleanser, one with the right mixture of ingredients and absence of toxic ones. In the next chapter we will go into detail of your options.

You don't want to wash away the good with the bad. Imagine waxing your car for 10 straight hours with sand paper and Ajax. Be sure that there will be no more shine on that vehicle. Just like this you can wash away the natural oils produced by your skin. As soon as you get out of the shower take a few minutes and apply a soothing moisturizing ointment.

Dressing right, like layering in the winter, and sun protection in the summer, will render dividends.

Inflammation is a common variable in all forms of eczematous skin; therefore the cream we choose must also combat the infiltration of inflammatory cells in the skin.

Chapter Eight
Acne, Rosacea and Age Spots

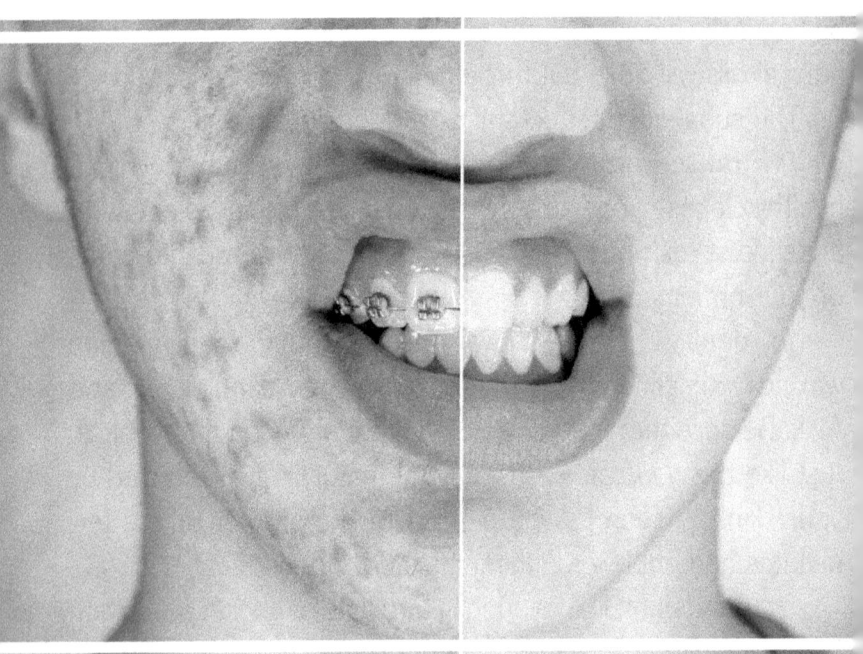

Pimples and pimples on older people

Oh those dreaded days of youth spent popping, squeezing, hiding those pustule ugly bumps on our face. Can you believe that they can come back again later!!

Acne is such an important and overwhelming problem, that it will be impossible to cover this topic in depth in this book. It is however possible to lay out the basic facts and suggest ways to deal with the problem. Rosacea is the continuation of the same problem into the later years in life.

No longer worried about what the kids in school will think about you, but still concerned about how you look.

For the most part, acne and rosacea are inflammations at the base of hair follicles extending to involve surrounding structures. Inflammation is categorized, generally, into chronic and acute inflammation. Basically this means old or new inflammation. Each has a different predominant cell type and presentation. In skin, lymphocytes can be observed in the dermis or epidermis, and are there as a response to different stimuli. Their job is to attack and protect on a cellular level. They appear to defend any further destruction of the microscopic elements in any part of the body.

When tissue is actually destroyed or beyond repair the acute inflammatory cells finish the job and are the reason for pus or pustules.

The entire process in the case of acne and rosacea has a certain order to it. First there is a stimulus, then a cell reaction.

Eventually a tiny area is beyond repair, eaten away by a different type of inflammatory cell, and then expelled out of the body through a pustule on the surface.

Just like everything else about the body, the reason for change and decay has several factors. First there are your genes which for the most part determine the type of skin you have. In the case of pimples, diet and stress play a huge role.

We all have the common experience of breaking out during exams, or a first date. In earlier chapters we discussed the tiny nerve endings in the skin which transmit and receive information.

High stress is like a constant electric signal pounding away at every cell. Like noise during a concert doesn't let you fully appreciate the music, well constant stress inhibits your body from normal functions.

The skin needs constant attention on every level. Your body has its own cellular defense structures working at maintaining the status quo. We each are obliged to make smart decisions about our diet, soaps and general life style.

I remember my grandmother warning against too much chocolate or greasy food, was she right? Today there is no real proof establishing a direct link between chocolate and pimples, but there is proof that fatty foods can make those with the tendency towards pimples get more and bigger bumps.

There are places on this planet where the natives don't even have a word for pimple, like New Guinea. But there is proof that when the natives of Papua are exposed to typical western fast foods, the first impact the modern world has on them is the new word, pimple.

By studying the diet of those people never affected by pimples we can make certain assumptions.

Fatty substances have an interesting role in the appearance and resolution of acne and rosacea. The Chinese have ancient formulations which use fatty acid mixtures found in plant oil as a principle ingredient in topical creams.

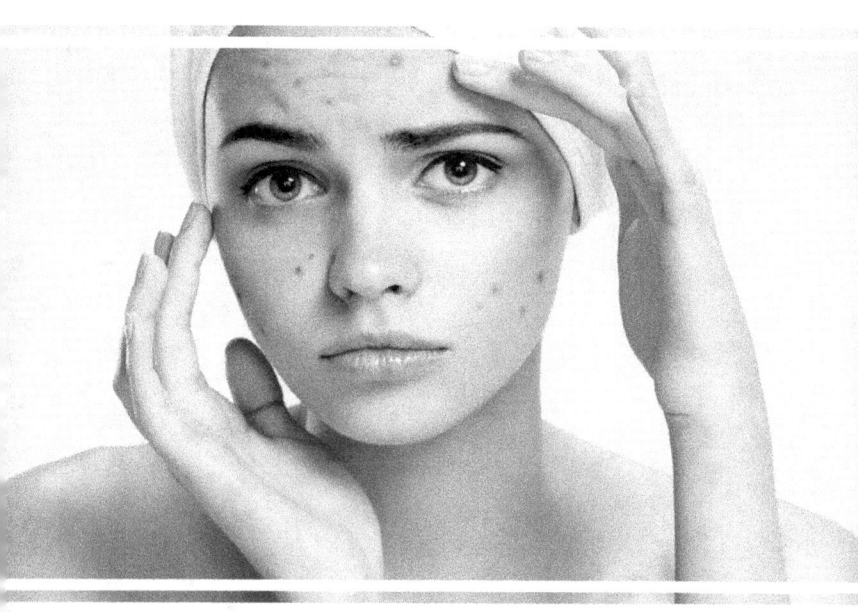

The avoidance of many foods along with the addition of new and healthier variants has a definitive positive influence on the appearance and duration of pimples.

The treatment of the inflammation of the skin is important. Aspirin or salicylic acid along with benzoyl peroxide can be beneficial. There are dermatologists that recommend antibiotics and stronger anti-inflammatory agents like hydrocortisone used topically as a remedial agent for pimples.

There are more aggressive methods to attack the long-term damage accrued by a life time of poping zits. Laser treatments, peals, exfoliate with application of topical ointment.

Whether you have eczema, acne or rosacea the approach is the same; understand your tendencies by knowing your skin type. Then make every conscious decision to protect, avoid and minimize.

Age Spots

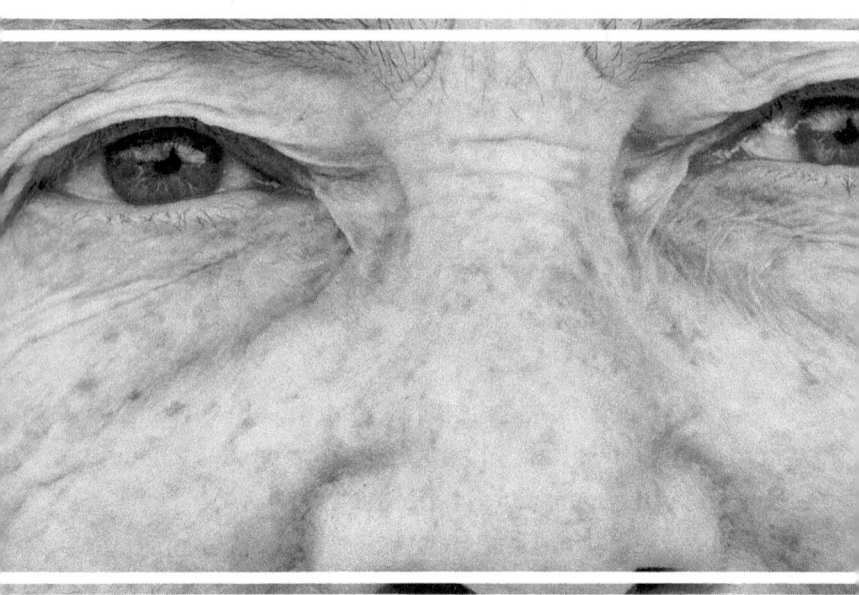

Another worrisome apparition of age is unwanted spots, colors laid out in patches of plain or lumpy lesions. The appearance of pigmented areas should never be taken lightly. The types of markings we will address in this chapter are commonly referred to as liver spots or aging spots. These markings are benign, or not clinically significant, just a blemish. As we grow older a vigilant attitude to watch out for dangerous lesions of the skin, that if detected quickly are cured with minor surgical procedures.

Liver spots are non-elevated light to dark brown and most commonly seen on the face and arms, you guessed it, sun exposed areas of your body. There really is no medical treatment required, but they are a sore spot to the careful observer. Like so many other terms referring to the skin, this is just another misnomer. The spots and your liver function are completely unrelated. Does the appearance of the spots bother you? Than there are remedies to this nuisance.

Have you ever noticed that some pregnant woman develop a pigmented face, well this is called melisma; and actually very similar to age spots, a.k.a. liver, spots, brown spots, sun spots. The pigment in your skin is produced by the melanocytes, which can be found in the base of the superficial covering of the skin, the epidermis. Whether your African or Anglo, both have the same number of melanocytes. It is the amount and location of the pigment, which make the visual qualitative difference.

When a new spot occurs you should watch it. Look at the borders, are they regular or jagged? Is it elevated? Has it changed in appearance?

There are those pigmented areas that have been lingering around since childhood. Like Nevi, or birthmarks. Also freckles come and go depending on the extent of sun exposure. If within or from of these long time companions, there begins to develop a new and bigger pigmented area, you should go see your doctor immediately. Perhaps a biopsy is warranted to rule out a malignancy, like melanoma. Most cancers of the skin are completely cured by a local wide excision, but the melanoma warrants quick and aggressive attention.

There are so many creams and natural remedies on the market that claim to eliminate age spots. The best choice is to consult a professional for proper guidance.

In the last few years there has been much controversy over the skin pigmentation of the late and great Michael Jackson, and also the baseball player Sammy Sosa.

These African American celebrities slowly became whiter and whiter. Speculation abounds as to how this is possible. From the camp of the celebrities they speak of a disease called vitiligo, which is the loss of pigmentation.

The reason for the variance of color over the years was a cause of great controversy and to my knowledge has never been clearly dealt with. In any case there are methods to bleach or discolor areas of unwanted pigment.

Age spots begin to appear around the age of forty. We talked about the slow regeneration of cells at later years, and the constant turnover of new cells. As we grow older our metabolism slows down, and in come the wrinkles, dots and spots.

Like an unwanted guest we immediately think of ways to stick around and have them leave.

Several new methods to deal with these aging problems are currently available.

While you're looking for a solution take shelter in what you already know, protect your skin from the sun as much as possible. Use the right clothing and sun blocks.

There are age-old remedies like Vitamin A, now synthetic components like retinoid regulate the growth ratios of our individual skin cells.

Most dermatologists agree that alpha hydroxyl acids work to break up the superficial skin summetry, the keratin layer of the epidermis, allowing them to hit the road and slough away.

Follow the yellow brick road. We started our trip chit chatting about your worries and learning about what skin is, and what it's made of.

The epidermis is a constantly changing mesh of layered epithelial cells, all bound together. Within the framework are nerve endings, melanocytes, protein and fatty fluid all flowing within a lake of salty water.

The melanin is made in the bottom, but deposited all over the deeper layers of epidermis. Those cells grow old and rise like the smoke from a fire, leaving a tainted residual image in whatever is left after the cell dies, the keratin on the surface. Our target is this superficial layer, and here there are choices to make.

My suggestion is no different from any other problem to confront. First try a conservative approach, and see if it works. If however the initial assessment or future unresponsiveness is clearly evident, then you must resort to more aggressive strategies.

First avoid the sun, and wash away unwanted color, but always be vigilant.

If you have light skin, and have waited away countless hours at the beach and tanning booth, be ready to deal with the consequences.

There are bleaching creams that are prescription if in higher concentrations, and non-prescription with lower concentrations. All contain hydroquinone with retinoid and steroids. (Hydroquinone is known to be VERY VERY BAD for the skin and BANNED IN EUROPEAN COUNTRIES)

A whole series of alternatives follow from laser to cryotherapy, and onto dermabrasion. These should only be done under a physician's care.

Again why not opt for a less aggressive method first. It might take a bit longer, but creams with glycolic acid, hydroquinone and kojic acid show promising results.

Chapter Nine
The Rocky Raccoon, Black Eyes and Circle

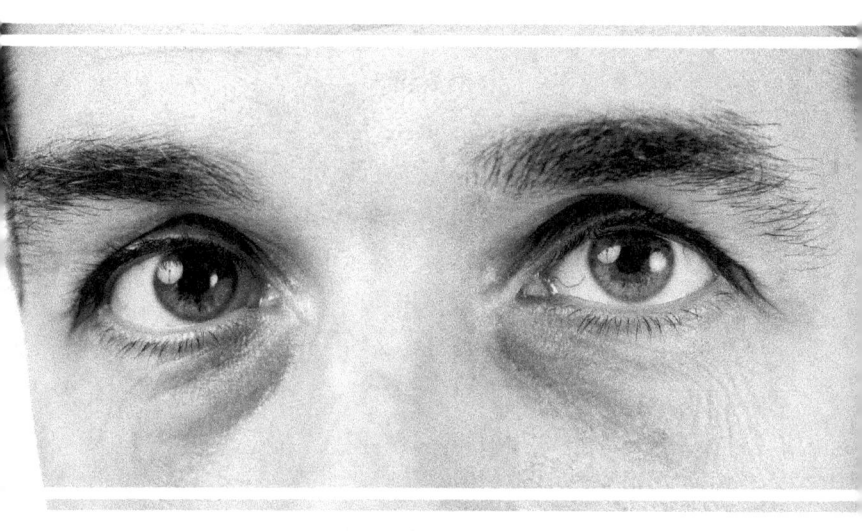

"Are you tired or just getting old?"
Rocky Raccoon

"Hey buddy, Were you up all night?" This is a nosy person wondering why those black circles are under your eyes. Black circles can be present at any age because of illness, fatigue and sometimes even allergies. Aging can bring on black circles to last longer and arise easier. In any event there are several cures.

There are as many physiologic reasons for black circles as there are cures. The epidermis is very thin in this area and vascular and pigment alterations are easily visible. Like a very thin curtain, what's going on behind the scene is readily seen.

If you're a hardcore party animal the circles could be a fashion statement, but for the most part they give one a sickly and tired appearance, to say the least.

In younger individuals the causes include genetic predisposition, heavy alcohol intake and smoking. Perhaps nasal congestion or gluten intolerance could be the cause. If you are in your forties and fifties and never had black circles so quickly formed, than the cause is thin skin and visible blood vessels due to less fatty tissue in the area.

A natural remedy should always be tried first. Be as cool as a cucumber, and slice on thinly, but be sure it was in your freezer for a while. Lay back and dream, and let your puffy eyes simmer down. A slice over each eye every day for 15 minutes will work wonders.

Every cougar knows this trick. While researching for this chapter it was astonishing how many home remedies people swear by. I am only including the ones that I can testify to.

1. Cold caffeine, in tea bags left over night in refrigerated water works wonders. Take the time to lay down in the morning after rising and before getting on with your day. The cold caffeine constricts the small vessels underlying the per orbital region, allowing the fluid accumulated in the extracellular tissue to ease back into the circulatory system. Thus the puffing goes down much like a diuretic effect.

2. Tilt your head back put some salty nose drops in your nose and cold teabags on your eyes.

3. There are more desperate and quicker remedies that have astonishing results, but they are too short lived. One is the cold steak, which is just gross, who wants a dead carcass on their face.

The other is a freezing spoon; this is too much like a boxers cure for a bloody nose.

4. There is something quite pleasant that seems to have great results. Go to sleep baby!

5. Stop drinking alchohol like a fish, and let your dreams abound.

Now take the time to look at your general health and diet. There we go again, back to Rome.

If you want to have a vivid realization take a trip to an alcoholic rehab facility, as a volunteer I hope, and take a gander at the patients that come walking through the door on by one. Then stop back a week later and check them out a gain. Nutrition rest and detoxification are the key elements to getting over the hump of an abusive life style. The point is, once a healthy diet replaces the intoxicants the dark circles seem to vanish. Even Houdini would be impressed by the vanishing act.

Chapter Ten
Puffy Eyes

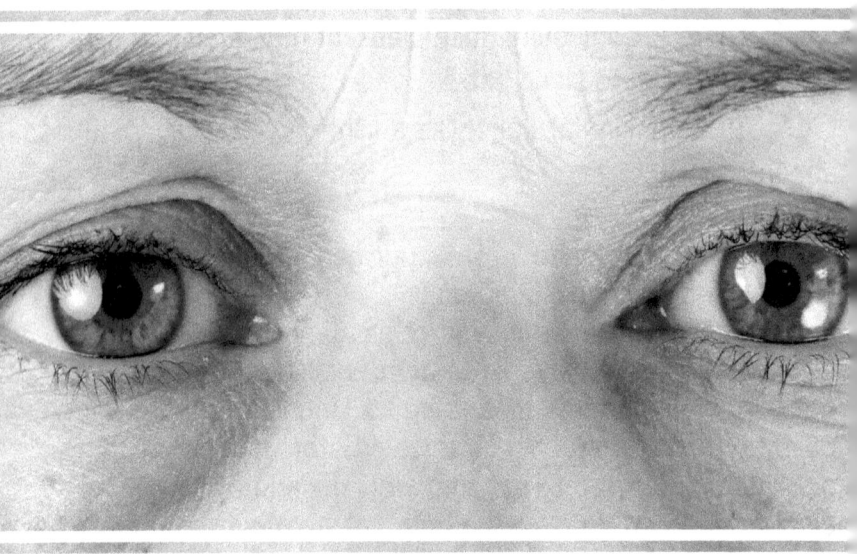

Puffy eyes mean too much liquid in a small area. The combination of superficial vessels, fluid moving out of the vessel and into the subcutaneous tissue. By decreasing the salt intake, and increasing Vitamin K and B-12 we take rapid steps towards flushing out the unwanted fluid buildup. What do dark circles, party animals, sickly people and oldies but goodies have in common? Malnutrition. So eat healthy, stop poring poison into your body, at least for a while. After utilizing all the natural and logical remedies, step it up. Make yourself pretty again. Take the time to research all the creams available, whether they are rejuvenation components, camouflage or night remedies; use the entire arsenal available.

If you quit smoking, eat more vegetables, relax a little and enjoy yourself, those black circles will go away. If this motherly advice is just too much, go buy some sunglasses and wear them all night long.

In the chapters that follow we will discuss our favorite ingredients which must be present in the creams you choose.

We will also take a holistic approach to handle the aging process.

You can't turn back the hands of time, but you can role with the punches.

Beautiful skin and thus, an attractive appearance are much more complicated than what meets the eye. What is reflected on the skin surface is the culmination of many factors like; healthy diet and subsequent nutrients to fuel the metabolic process.

Remember our previous discussions about the histologic make-up of the skin. Each underlying layer and the tiny structures like elastin, sweat glands; all play a role in the outer semblance of the skin. Let's not forget other hidden denominators like exercise and mental attitude, whose combined effect should never be underestimated.

Skin Sagging

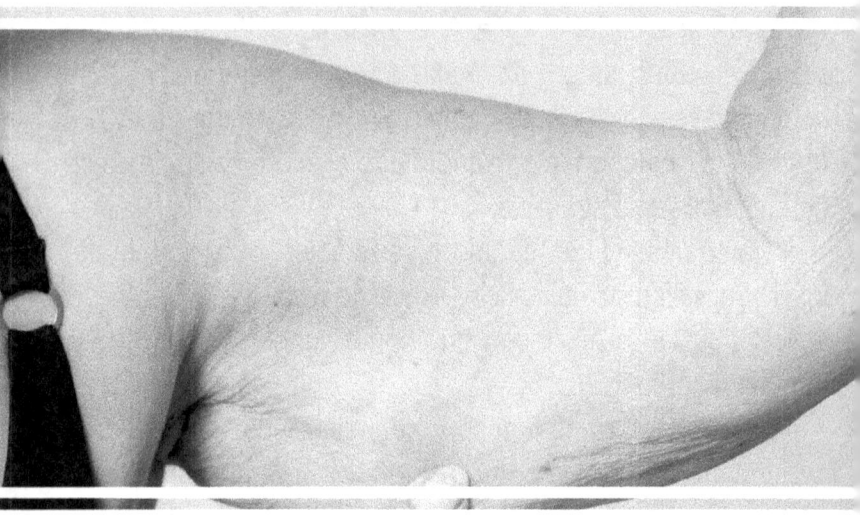

Take sagging skin. This is seen as an outer drooping of the skin surface.

The real problem lies beneath the surface. Depending on your facial bone structure and strength of fibro muscular attachments to the osseous tissue, the deep cushion on which the skin lies begins to loosen.

At the same time the dermal fibro connective tissue becomes weak with normal wear and tear effects, the outer skin is actually being held up, stretched out and tightened by the subcutaneous components.

So when we see sagging skin, realize that the skin sags because of the loss of the supporting structures. The mental picture which comes to mind is a beautiful classic ballet dancer being held high in the air by a strong companion.

The eyes of the entire audience are fixed on the graceful girl; few notice the tense strong boy holding her up. The boy is the underlying strength, which allows the girls beauty to be seen.

Thinning Skin

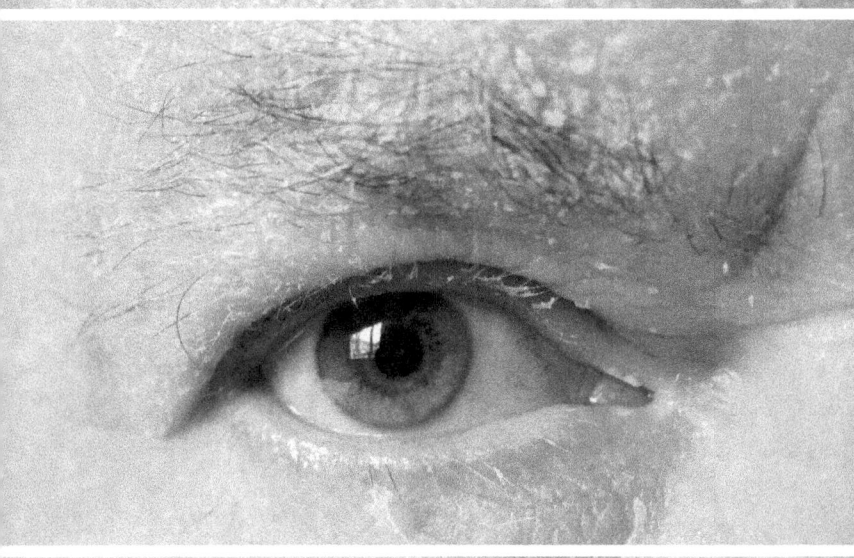

The example of thinning skin allows us to see a glimpse of what is really happening. Thinning skin is a normal part of the aging process. As we grow older the cellular turnaround is not as quick. We discussed how epithelial cells are born, live and die.

As the cycle of birth continues the multilayered epidermis remains intact, the cells do not regenerate as fast, and the predominant layer is the cellular superficial keratin surface. Now there is a thin transparent curtain where a much thicker and protective shield used to be.

Now the underlying tiny blood vessels become visible, as the gathering of previously unseen pigments in the dermal epidermal junction.

Isn't it amazing that when you picture a hero, or favor a particular movie star, they always look very beautiful or handsome as the case may be? Have you ever imagined a hero to be ugly? Off course not. The good guy is always a looker, and the bad one is just plain ugly.

According to numerous scientific studies and plain old commonsense there is little doubt if you are better looking you will most likely land the job before a brighter but homely applicant. Who gets the boyfriend, the pretty or ugly sister? Once again, chances are the pretty sister. Even Cinderella – every woman's perfect fairytale - before she found the magic shoes was basically beautiful… she just needed those shoes to spread her wings and get all dolled up.

In the surface layer of skin there are tiny nerves which act as receptors and transmit perceptions of touch - cold, hot, sensual or not. These are the nerves, which connect with a highly complex intelligent network, far more sophisticated than the latest computer software.

All of our sense organs, eyes, ears, nose, mouth and skin; are constantly transmitting information through the nerves attached to the central and peripheral nervous system. The result is a conglomeration of data that has to be processed. We have spent a lifetime gathering information just so that an opinion can be made. So we already have a personal concept of beauty. That picture is tainted with cultural and popular influences. In general most people from a common region will agree on what is beautiful, and what is plain ugly.

Remember the epidermis is paper thin, and underneath the protein support structures, laden with glands; the dermis. Finally the skin insulation, the subcutaneous fatty tissue. With time the effects of the sun, gravity and poisons we ingest, take their toll.

When I was a kid the images of dessert nomads wearing these long white robes, and covering their entire body made for mysterious images. When I was 12 years old my aunt brought me on a trip to the Mojave desert in southern north America. It was 104 degrees in the middle of June, not a tree in sight. The first time I was exposed to this sun the vision of these dessert nomads came to mind. I was in a pair of shorts, and immediately took my shirt off to cool off. How could those dudes in the dessert survive with all those clothes on? Boy did I learn my lesson the hard way. Within minutes I was sunburned and quite uncomfortable. Soon my head was wrapped with my t-shirt, and body covered with anything so that the sun could not burn my flesh. This is lesson number one. Learn from those who know how to protect themselves from the sun. The sun is a double-edged sword. We can't live without it, but we must protect ourselves from too much exposure. The lessons in medicine seemed to be learned too late. There is a common joke at medical conventions that describes the different specialists. The Internal Medicine doctor knows about everything, but doesn't do much of anything, except tell you to take few aspirins and call in the morning. The surgeon, well he is willing to do anything at all, but he doesn't understand much of anything; when in doubt, cut it out. Then there's the pathologist. He knows about everything, is willing and able to do anything, one problem, he's always too late.

A wise man said that an ounce of prevention is worth a pound of cure. This must have been the father of preventative medicine. It makes perfect sense that if you are careful enough to understand the dangers around you, and realize that no one is exempt from injury or disease, perhaps we would take much more care of our body, soul and mind.

With the thinning of aging skin come the purging rays of sunshine within. Ultraviolet radiation shears apart the matrix of collagen and elastin. The damage causes the formation of wrinkles as well as visibility of vascular structures, and irregular production and absorption of pigment. Add to this little dermal structures producing fewer secretions to keep our surface moist, and what do you get? Dry, scaly skin with spots, red blots and wrinkles in between. The changes become evident in the forties, but are ever present in the fifties.

Moisture, exfoliation are welcomed to speed up the dead cell turnover ratio.

Perhaps the foremost authority in the world on skin lesions and the underlying physiopathology is Dr. Bernard Ackerman. Every dermatologist on the planet has one of his books on his shelf. His depth of knowledge includes an empathetic understanding of how many physicians and lay people categorize skin lesions. In his book 'Histologic Diagnosis of Inflammatory Skin Diseases", an entire section is dedicated to confusing terms. Just think that if doctors are often confused with the manner of description, terminology and cause of many skin lesions, how the normal citizen with a sincere interest to learn and deal with aging skin can be spaced out by the influx of so much new knowledge. This is not a book intended for physicians or skin specialists, though we do offer an educational course for those that which to understand the microscopic changes observed in diseases of the skin.

Chapter Eleven
Role with punches,
Skin issues with Aging

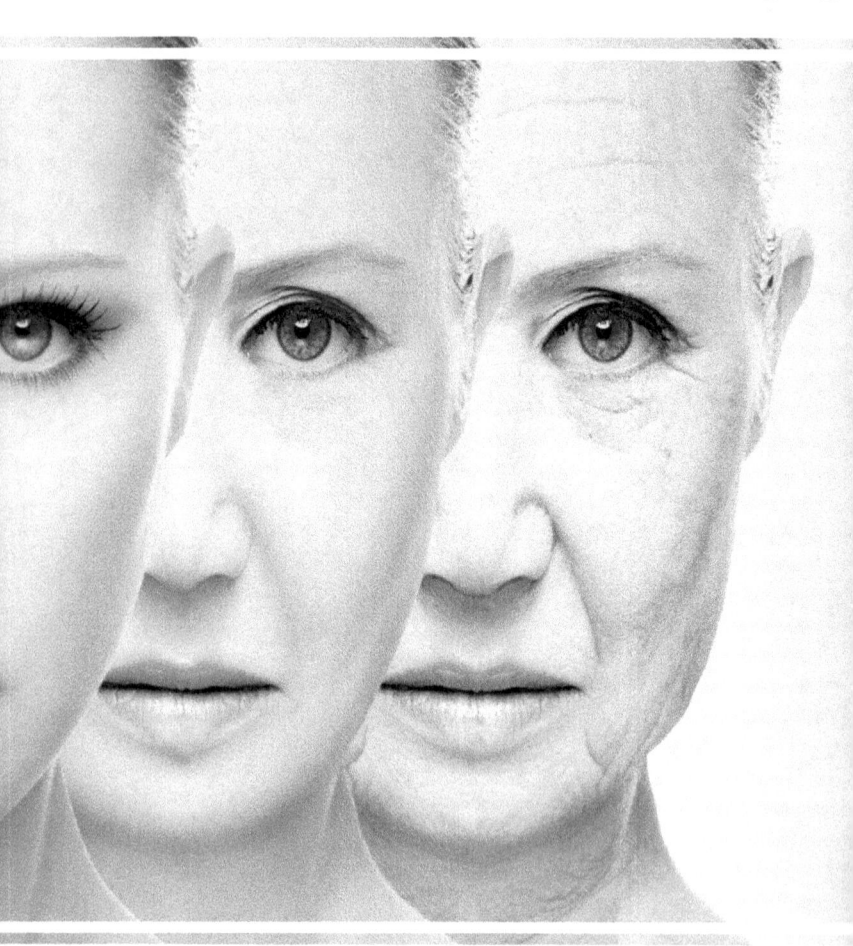

The clock is ticking and calendar months progressing. "If I could turn back the hands of time." No matter how pure your diet, or degree of tranquility achieved, the wear and tear that comes along with aging will manifest. Every organ begins to change, loosing elasticity and signs of diminished functional capacity become evident. We must accept the changes as the natural course, but you don't have to sit back and watch the show.

Before we discuss the ways to minimize the effects of aging on the skin, you should have a basic understanding of the terms and description of each complication. That way the method of treatment is an informed personal choice. There are certain things that just are, like your genetic make-up. Your genes are yours forever, no altering that, but the good news is that many other influences cause a negative spiral effect on early aging signs of the skin. One of the most blatant lies is "beauty is only skin deep." A close second is "beauty is in the eyes of the beholder." Of course this becomes true if you have severe visual problems. Beautiful features, like the distance between your eyes, or prominent cheek bones, are impossible to alter. Other things like sagging jaws and a droopy neck, or perhaps a small chin: can be improved with surgical techniques.

Small lips and many deep wrinkles can be erased with Botox or skin fillers, but we will concentrate on those lesions which are treated and improved with non-invasive techniques. We are interested in re plenishing or maintaining that natural glow. The semblance of health is no different than the reflection of happiness: one just appears to glow. This glow is a twofold

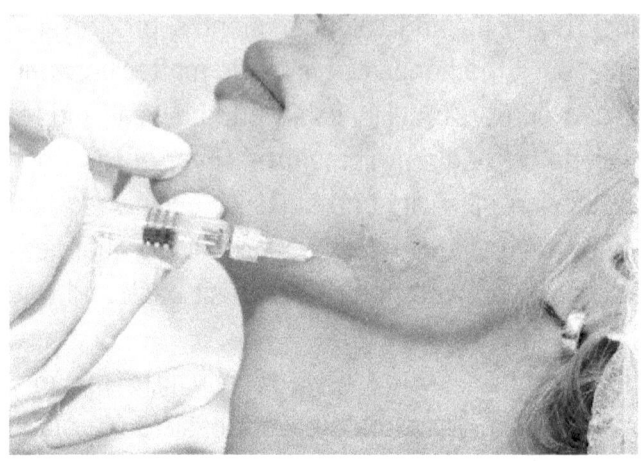

manifestation. It is the evidence of healthy diet and positive attitude, and it is also how you want your skin to be perceived.

Isn't it amazing that when you picture heroes, or favor particular movie stars, they always look very pretty. The good guy is always a looker, and the bad one is just plain ugly. Is there any doubt that if you are better looking you will most likely land the job before a brighter but homely competitor.

Who gets the boyfriend, the pretty or ugly sister?

There are two forms of images to consider, what others see, and what you see of yourself. Both are important. Our interest is to focus on an objective scenario, you; then consider how to improve the landscape. In the interim we must utilize the human hard drive, to process all the data.

In the surface layer of skin there are tiny nerves which act as receptors and transmit perceptions of touch. Cold, hot, sensual or not. These are the nerves which connect with a highly complex intelligent network, far more sophisticated than the latest computer software.

All of our sense organs, eyes, ears, nose, mouth and skin; are constantly transmitting information through the nerves attached to the central and peripheral nervous system. The result is a conglomeration of data that has to be processed. We have spent lifetime gathering information just so that an opinion can be made. So we already have a personal concept of beauty. That picture is tainted with cultural and popular influences. In general most people from a common region will agree on what is beautiful, and what is plane ugly.

There are cultural differences, but there are common denominators shared by any genetic or opinionated imprints.

Once the process of aging begins to show it's true colors, the result is deterioration of the microscopic elements in the dermis, the collagen and elastin, with gradual thinning of the outer layer of skin, the epidermis. Like the way termites slowly destroy a nice house. At first there is no sign of these tiny creatures eating away at the wood which keeps our home solid. They move into the ceiling beams, walls, closets, and are persistently hacking away at whatever is around. For so long only an expert can notice their presence. Eventually the damage is visible to the naked eye. Even at late stages there are solutions. The only difference is that the action needed to restore the original appearance needs to be more drastic.

In the face we are looking for that natural glow, the expression of health and vigor.

Beauty is always a two way street. Inner spiritual and organic health is represented by a shiny and firm skin tone. What do you see in the mirror? Is it your soul or liver? Can you see the vitamins flowing through the blood and into each cell? If you can make sure you don't step on your cape as you fly out the window superman or wonder woman. If your skin is glowing, it makes you feel better. So the energy is bidirectional. Pretty on the inside, see it on the outside.

If you can't see it, maybe there is a reparative process that will have to do at first.

Your skin is the ambassador of your body. It's only proper that the best possible impression must be our only objective.

In the early chapters we discussed the structure and functions of the skin.

Remember the epidermis is paper thin, and underneath the proteinaceous support structures, laden with glands; the dermis, and finally the skin insulation, the subcutaneous fatty tissue. With time the effects of the sun, gravity and poisons we ingest take their toll.

When I was a kid the images of dessert nomads wearing these long white robes, and covering their entire body made for mysterious images. When I was 12 years old my aunt brought me on a trip to the Mojavedesert in southern north America. It was 104 degrees in mid-June, not a tree in site. The first time I was exposed to this sun the vision of these dessert nomads came to mind. I was in a pair of shorts, and immediately took my shirt off to cool off. How could those dudes in the dessert survive with all those clothes on? Boy did I learn my lesson the hard way. Within minutes I was sunburned and quite uncomfortable. Soon my head was wrapped with my t shirt, and body covered with anything so that the sun could not burn my flesh. This is lesson number one. Learn from those who know how to protect you from the sun. The sun is a double edged sword. We can't live without it, but we must protect ourselves from too much exposure.

The lessons in medicine seemed to be learned too late. There is a common joke at medical conventions that describes the different specialists. The Internal Medicine doctor knows about everything, but doesn't do much of anything, except tell you to take few aspirins and call in the morning. The surgeon, well he is willing to do anything at all, but he doesn't understand much of anything; when in doubt, cut it out. Than there's the pathologist. He knows about everything, is willing and able to do anything, one problem, he's always too late.

A wise man said that an ounce of prevention is worth a pound of cure. This must have been the father of preventative medicine. It makes perfect sense that if you are careful enough to understand the dangers around you, and realize that no one is exempt from injury or disease, perhaps we would take much more care of our body, soul and mind.

With the thinning of aging skin comes the purging rays of sunshine within. Ultraviolet radiation shears apart the matrix of collagen and elastin. The damage causes the formation of wrinkles as well as visibility of vascular structures, and irregular production and absorption of pigment. Add to these little dermal structures producing less secretion to keep our surface moist, and what do you get? Dry, scaly skin with spots, red blots and wrinkles in between.

The changes become evident in the forties, but are ever-present in the fifties.

Moisture, exfoliation are welcomed to speed up the dead cell turnover ratio.

Chapter Twelve
Love potion #9

"I held my nose, I closed my eyes, I took a drink."

No, this is not the way we roll. There is no fool proof method to achieve glowing skin, but there are wide arrays of ingredients that have a good track record in rendering dividends to obtain healthy epithelium.

An intelligent consumer will take the time to look at the ingredients of those skin products which publicly claim benefits. Many of the over the counter creams share common components as some prescription medications, only differing in concentration and formulation.

There are substances which have been used for hundreds of years as natural remedies passed from generation to generation. As scientific methods and equipment progress, so does the art and science of documenting biophysical effects, and direct correlations of natural remedies and subsequent cream formulations.

The goal is to create a skin cream with just the right percentage and binding of ingredients to have both a cosmetic and healing effect to deal with the process of aging. In this chapter we will discuss several ingredients which have demonstrated substantial benefit independently.

The order of the components is not important, and no one ingredient outweighs the usefulness of another. The objective of this chapter is to give the consumer the knowledge to choose the cream best suited for her/his type of skin, by understanding the active ingredients.

Recently esoteric research into stem cell utilization in skin creams has added a whole new twist to an ancient concern. Today we are looking at biochemical and genetic influence to catalyze the regeneration of new cells. Just as the relevance of every new clinical trial is taken into consideration when formulating a cream, so is the accumulated wisdom of every mentionable culture. Woman a thousand years ago were also concerned about their skin, and interesting enough natural remedies for dry skin, sun burn, wrinkles can be found in texts on every continent .

In this chapter we look at the key ingredients that you should look for in the cream you choose.

Many products will contain a varying number of the ingredients discussed, but each will vary in the mixture , content and formulation. Let's begin our tour into the secret world of skin care remedies.

Acmella Oleracea

Deep in the tropical jungles of Brazil, lays a miniscule yellow flower with a hat like red top.

For thousands of year local Indians seek the budding spectacular flower when suffering from tooth aches.

Chewing on this mysterious herb results in an immediate relief from the agonizing pain. Many have tried to identify

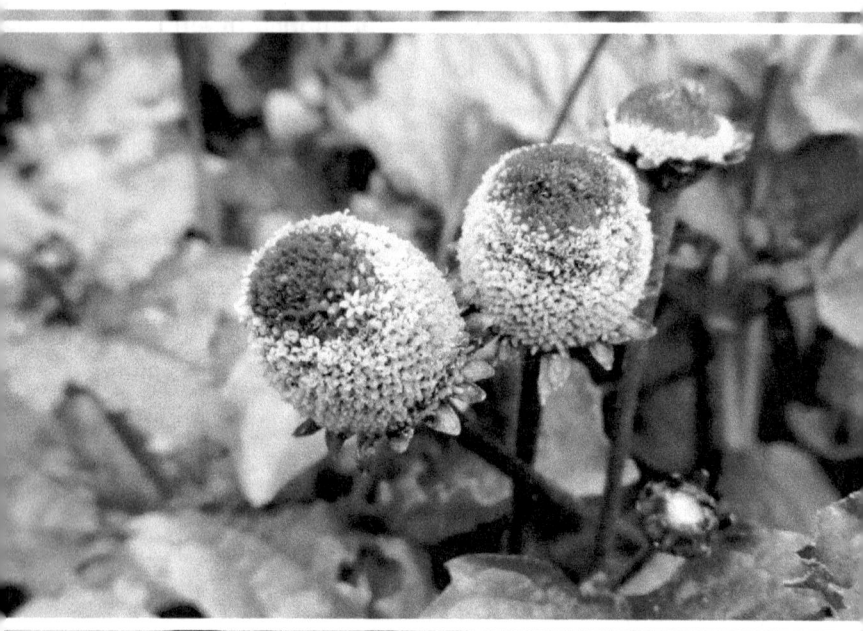

the actual biochemical compound with the medicinal effect, but no clear cut derivative has been identified, though we know it is an alkylamide similar to Spilanthol. This is what we do know. There is instant relaxation of the muscles around the mouth when chewed. This is a visible effect; you can actually see a relief of tension. Following this same line of reasoning, if you prepare a cream with Acmella Oleracea, the facial muscles which are contracted, accentuating wrinkles, will loosen, thus decreasing the facial lines around the mouth. This is simply an anatomic effect because there are more muscles around the mouth than any other region of the body.

In some circles this unique red and yellow flower can be referred to as 'jungle Botox', without the needle.

By the way if you happen to be in a jungle when using this ingredient it is an excellent mosquito repellant.

Retinol or Vitamin A

One of the most studied vitamins for skin products is vitamin A.

Retinol is derived from animals, eggs and purer forms come from carrots and spinach. The biochemical structure and pathways of synthesis are quite complex and an essential component of any graduate level class in biochemistry and pharmacology. Let me try my best to explain in laymen terms why retinol is an important component for the skin cream of choice.

As retinol is converted to different by products by natural reactions, each new variant has a benefit of its own. The skin, bones, stem cells and eyes all need Vitamin A to maintain health. Vitamin A was first synthesized two Dutch chemists just after the Second World War,

David Van Dorp and Josef Arens were responding to concerns of the scientific community for over 100 years to produce this vitamin to deal with the manifestations of its deficiency. Some of the problems were dry and scaling skin, visual difficulty and friable bone structure. We all have heard of the role of vitamin A in visual functions, but the non-visual functions are just as important. We know today that retinol plays a role in immunologic function, protecting us from infections. The reason it must be in your cream of choice is that scientists have shown that vitamin A stimulates cell turn over at the stem cell level. Remember our early description of this concept? If you increase the rate at which new skin cells are produced, the older cells slough off at a quicker pace.

Collagen synthesis is also stimulated thus giving the skin a fresh appearance. The result is both a cosmetic and medicinal effect when used topically. In the latter it is used for the treatment of acne and keratosis, an ugly bump in the skin seen after the age of 40.

So, make sure you see Retinol or Vitamin A on the skin cream list of active ingredients.

Shea Butter

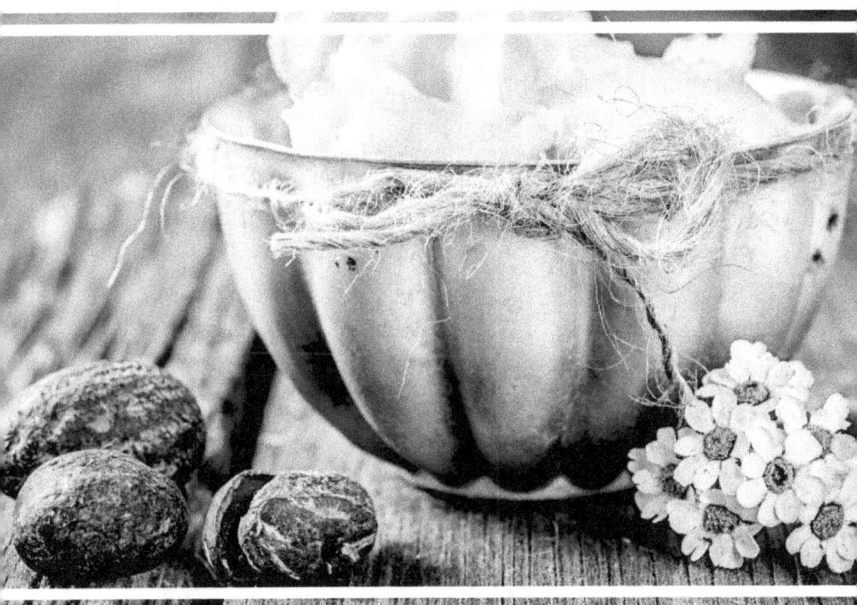

For centuries Africans have known the benefits of this natural oil for beautiful skin and hair. A secret which has been passed from generation to generation. The butter is made by grinding a unique nut that is born many years after the trees branches and flowers come into being. Many of these Shea-Karite trees take more than 15 years to reap the fatty laden nuts.

Like a vintage wine fermenting in a barrel, the oils inside the center of the nuts slowly evolve into a powerful fatty acid.

The natural preparation of butter from boiling the nuts has many proven benefits; from a natural moisturizer to relief of sunburn.

The oil restores the shiny appearance of healthy skin as well as the elasticity, by transporting high levels of vitamins A and E.

Vitamin E or Tocopherol is found in every single skin cream on the market. The reports verifying the positive effects of Vitamin E are well known to the public. The secret to optimal use in western countries is the method of preparation and delivery.

Ubiquinone or Coenzyme Q10

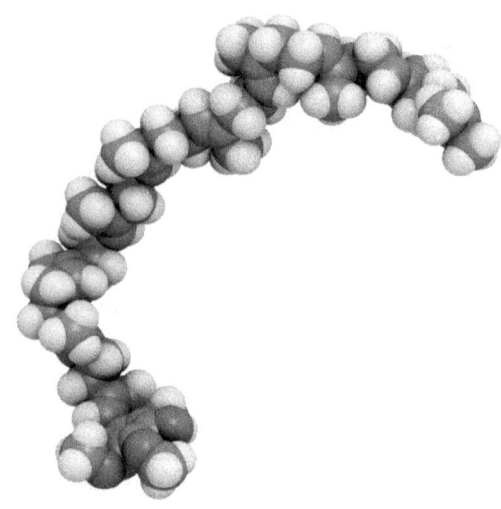

A breakthrough research project was conducted in 1999 and published by John T.A.Ely, Ph.D. and Cheryl A.Krone, Ph.D. in the journal of Orthomolecular Medicine. They proved that high levels of COQ10 slowed down the process of aging. The recommendation to supplement ubiquinone to reverse age related degradation was clearly made. In the 1970's this product was established as an important use to combat Congestive Heart Failure. CoQ10 works by generating energy in the form of ATP DE at the mitochondrial and also reducing cellular stress on the oxidative level.

Almost every proven formulation for an anti-aging cosmetic contains this particular coenzyme, and it is widely recognized already by the save European consumer.

In my research of 7 different products Proven to demonstrate improvement in age related skin manifestations, like wrinkles, age spots, pore enlargement; COQ10 was a persistent ingredient in each product. This fat soluble vitamin like substance is found in nearly every single cell , especially the epithelial skin cells, thus the origin of its name 'ubis' which means everywhere in latin. The oily isolated anti-oxidant finds its' way to the skins surface with the help of the tiny glandular sebaceous glands. These miniscule pumping dermal machines have ducts which lay sebum on the superficial layers of the epidermis.

Ubiquinone teams up with Vitamin E or Tocopherol to become the tag team kings of the anti-oxidation team. The shiny glistening surface of healthy skin is due to the presence of these skin surface fats, along with wax, cholesterol in a triglyceride or lipid base.

When I first started working on this book, my original working thesis was the concept of 'outer shield'. If you think about it, the skin is just like the armor knights use to wear into battle. The most vulnerable part of our body to chemicals in the ozone or polluted city air is the surface of the skin, just the place where you find the skin surface lipids. Similarly as the sun beats down on our leather surface, waiting for the insult and injury is CoEnzyme Q 10 or Ubiquinone. There it is, ready to lubricate and protect, with one minor problem; the supply is restricted with age. Elderly people practically have no COEQ10 left in the skin cells. So guess what, we have to replace it. The need to replenish the natural production pumped to the surface by the ducts of the sebaceous glands is also necessary after a good sunburn. The ultraviolet rays of the sun suck the skin dry of these fat soluble anti-oxidants.

Imagine an orange peel laid out on a sidewalk. Within minutes the shiny orange reflection turns into a dull brown glimmer less tint. The cracks become deeper and form grossly observable tracks. Just like this skin exposed to the sun quickly dries, shrivels and wrinkles. The Japanese learned the secrets of ubiquinone many years ago, and now it is considered an essential component of anti-aging skin cream.

Since it is a fact that ubiquinone is only second to Vitamin C as an essential nutrient, we should consider supplementing low levels, a natural occurrence with aging. Peter Langsjoen,MD is the author of the most important works describing the safety of replenishing ubiquinone. As we age we produce less, and irreversible damage can occur on a microscopic level that can speed up the already unstoppable aging process. Since there is overwhelming proof of the importance of ubiquinone in the prevention of age related degeneration, we must include this as an essential component in our recommendations'.

Glycine Soya or Soybean oil

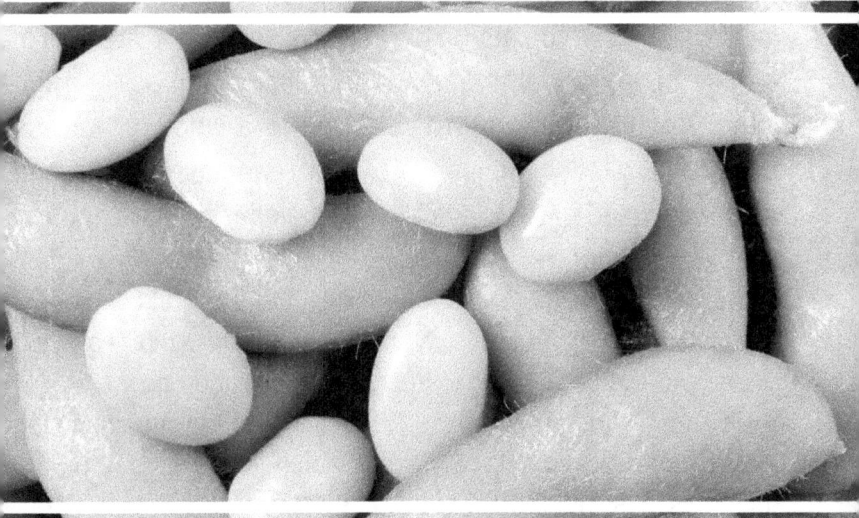

When mixing up the perfect cream you're going to add a lubricant. An oil, but not just any greasy film will do. Why not pick out natures' own super oil. It is common knowledge in the health conscious community of vegetarians and holistic crowds that soy products are the proteins of choice. By eliminating animal protein we immediately decrease the amount of free radicals in our system. By supplementing with soy we add an antioxidant to our regimen of health. So often we have referred to the negative effects of sun exposure and smoking on the skin. Well the underlying reason is the formation of free radicals which inhibit DNA synthesis and cell turnaround ratios. By doing so we inhibit the normal function of our immune system to combat infection and inflammation. According to recent literature, the use of antioxidants goes hand in hand with fighting the aging process. Now we are referring to a whole other use of natures' oil. For thousands of years woman in China and India have used oils on their skin as a cleanser, lubricant and a beauty solution.

Soya is not only a powerful antioxidant, but a vital component of any skin cream. You need a substance which will increase the viscosity of the potion, and act as a water retention agent. Soy oil or Glycine Soya is an emollient. A fancy way of saying something which when applied will retain the water in the center of the epidermis by sealing the pores with a viscous fatty layer.

Just like you can't bake a cake without butter or oil, no lotion is complete without a bit of this natural nutritious fatty acid called Glycine Soya or soybean oil. By itself will make your skin soft and smooth, combined with the other favorites of 'love potion # 9' it is a sure winner

The Palmitoyl family

Sometimes you have to get creative, literally. It's easy to think in terms of just replenishing what is missing, like adding a little oil to your engine when its' running a quart low.

Yet the possibility of stimulating production of things lost in time is also a good idea. There are ways of playing tricks on nature to get your way.

Have you ever stopped to think how birth control pills work? When a woman takes 'the pill' she is sending an artificial signal to the brain, telling the main computer that she is pregnant.

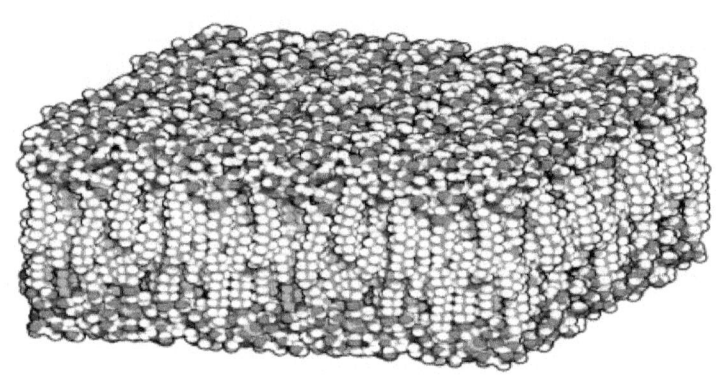

Actually her desire is to avoid pregnancy and she is able to accomplish this by ingesting a pill that causes the hypothalamus (or central control center) to diminish the secretion of hormones which stimulate the formation and release of follicles capable of being impregnated.

The body has many such trigger mechanisms and the skin has several hidden mechanisms designed with pinpoint accuracy to make sure those adequate supplies of nutrients, support and moisturizers are always available.

In nature, problems occur when these mechanisms cease to function with the same efficiency as intended.

In several previous references we have described how wrinkles are formed, and laid down the basic elements which make up the skin support structure, let me refresh your memory.

Fibroblasts are tiny cells located in the dermis which actually produce the collagen and elastin that form the micro skeletal support system of the skin.

The tent poles, remember? There are peptides in the circulation, specifically Palmitoyl oligopeptide which are actually fragments of degrading collagen.

One of the better known variants in this family is called Dermaxyl.

There is evidence that this compound is actually able to recruit cells to police damaged areas of skin. Like giving a jump start to an age or insult related slowing down of tissue repair,

Dermaxyl boosts the genetic expression of certain proteins(GCP, or Granulocytic Chemotactic Protein). Once the level of PAL begins to rise the body is aware that we need more collagen.

There are products available like Strivectin, which combine peptides with niacin for a significant boost in fibroblatic production of collagen.

In other words these products directly stimulate the ongoing cellular regeneration, or rejuvenation, by jump starting the cell turn around ratios.

The whole benefit of using peptides in combination with vitamins, antioxidants and oils; is to maintain and support a healthy skin barrier.

The long term effect is to provide extra support and tensile strength. This in turn will make wrinkles virtually disappear by increasing the thickness of the skin.

So this kicks off a sequence of events that cause an increase in the production of new collagen. If we link the entire chain of events, here's what happens.

Aging collagen begins to degrade

1. Palmitoyl oligopeptide is released into the dermis

2. A signal goes off saying, "hey body we need more collagen"

3. The fibroblasts are pushed into overdrive and produce fresh collagen

4. Wrinkle formation is reduced and even reversed

Bottom line, look for this ingredient when choosing your cream.

The benefits of Palmitoyl oligopeptides have been well documented as not only beneficial in treatment of wrinkles, but also unwanted pigment.

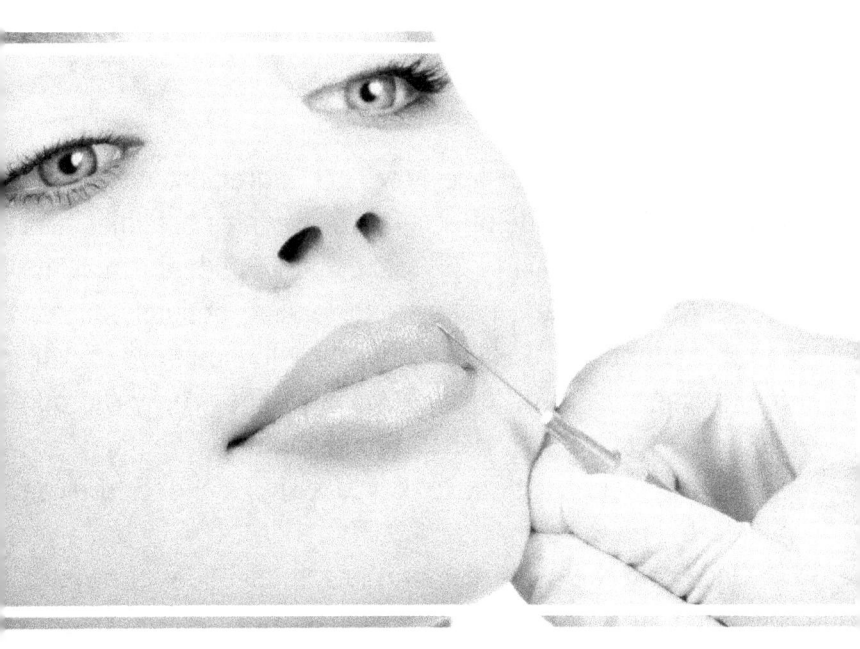

Dipeptide-2

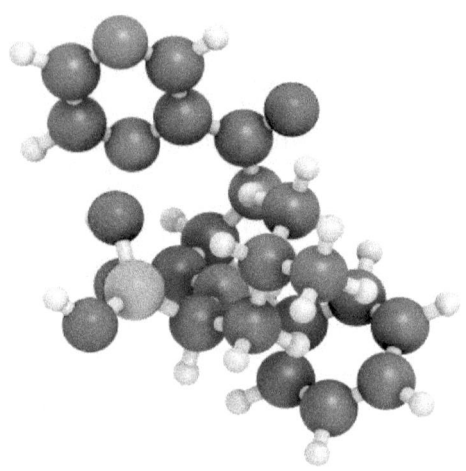

Up to now you can see how each ingredient mentioned adds a particular mode of action in delivering a healthier skin.

Two standard amino acids make up Dipeptide-2. On all the shelves of the cream, lotions, and tanning potions you can find this ingredient. It is most commonly found in eye creams due to many claims of a rapid combat of the "rocky raccoon syndrome", puffy dark rings around the eyes. Peptides are protein fragments that due to their size shape and texture can penetrate into the skin.

Once past the protective barriers the peptides can reach the prime target, fibroblasts. Remember our basic discussion of cell elements of the skin. Well it is the fibroblast which has the task of making the collagen that the skin needs. The collagen in turn provides the fortitude that the skin needs to stretch it out and avoid the early formation of wrinkles.

All skin creams with proven track records will contain peptides, dipeptides, and oligo-peptides in combination with an array of other vitamins, moisturizers, elasticizers.

The structure of the dipeptide will create a natural moisturizing effect.

The term Natural Moisturizing Factor is often used in the ever popular cream lingo pseudoscientific community.

Articles written to describe why anti-aging creams work are often miss leading and filled with unsubstantiated claims.

When we described some natural remedies to puffy eyes, like cold teabags, we failed to mention how this method works. Well common sense, if you have some basic physiology in your repertoire, tells us that when there is less than optimal lymphatic circulation, there tends to be regional edema.

This is another way of saying puffiness. So, if the lymphatic circulation is improved, then the regional puffiness will diminish. In my research I was unable to find a single scientific pre- clinical study to prove this in skin cream usage.

What is certain is that the structure of Dipeptide-2 is very similar to the fatty portion of the epidermis, thus its presence will help keep the water retention portion or lipid content enhanced. The result is that the moisture stays in the epidermis. This is one way to preserve the armor, the outer shield, thus protecting us from external irritants which cause dermatitis.

There is certainly enough proof that warrants throwing a little Dipeptide into the potion.

Vitamin C

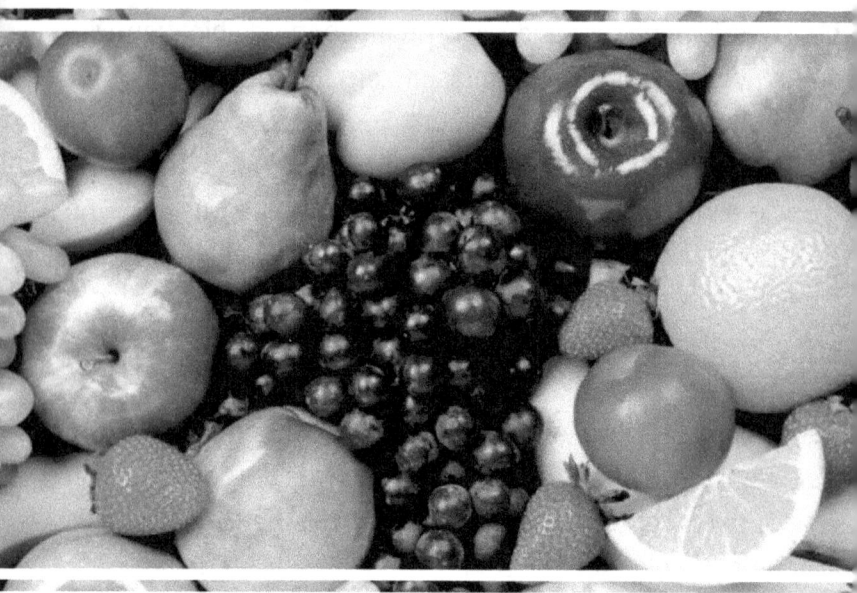

You cannot have a cream without vitamin C; might as well not even think about purchasing a healthy skin cream if there is no Vitamin C in it. If there is one ingredient that is unanimously seen as the most effective, it's vitamin C and derivatives. By derivatives, are compounds built from the base ingredient as Vitamin C.

Just as there is no doubt as to the effectiveness of vitamin C, it is clear how quickly the vitamin becomes unstable and ineffective. That's why the newer derivatives, like ascorbyl palmitate, are so important. Stability of an ingredient assures that it will actually live up to its potential. Sometimes a preclinical laboratory experiment will prove beyond a doubt that, in a test tube, there is an immediate boost of collagen production by fibroblasts when infused with ascorbic acid (Vitamin C).

The problem is that when you deal in a real life scenario, the exposure of vitamin C to the air will cause rapid oxidation and the subsequent formation of dangerous free radicals. The most successful use of vitamin C comes only after figuring a way out to make it more stable. The bad news is that this process is very expensive, driving way up the cost of the creams which include slowly oxidizing variants of Vitamin C.

Science has found a way to formulate vitamin C derivatives to be less irritating and more intrusive into the skin. Once you get the stabile vitamin C derivative like ascorbyl palmitate absorbed into the skin immediate effects are readily documented. The most important is the boost in collagen synthesis.

Be sure to buy fresh cream. Have you ever drunk old orange juice? Bitter, and not good for you. Well creams should be kept under the right temperature and used before expiration, or they will do more harm than good. A dead giveaway is a yellow tincture and topical irritation.

Keep your eye out for the latest formulations which include ascorbic acid combined with another acid like palmitate or phosphate.

Chapter Thirteen
Skin Types

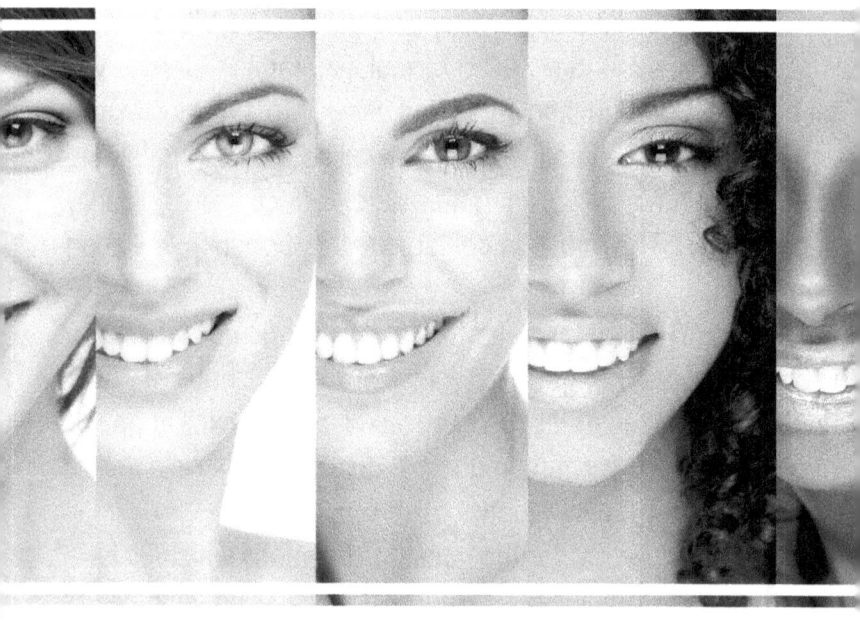

The Master Key to Solving Your Skin Issues

Skin Type: Simply, skin type is the description and interpretation of how and why your skin looks feels and behaves at it does. The huge benefit of knowing your skin type is having the master-key to fixing your different skin care problems. Not knowing your skin type is like trying to shoot for bull's eye in the dark.

In a previous chapter we discussed the parts of the skin and how we end up looking old based on how different layers of the skin play-out as we age.

In this chapter we'll identify your skin type so we can determine a customized solution for your specific skin aging issue. You see different skin types require different product formulations and different treatments.

No matter what race, age or gender, we all share the common structure and function of the skin. However, depending on our skin type the "solutions" to our skin aging varies. This chapter is actually a dialogue between you and me. I would like us to walk down a path together, leading you towards the realization of what skin type you have so you can take a customized approach for your skin.

It's fascinating how the same ingredients produce so many variants. Just like the mixture of the same spices and herbs in different percentages make completely different flavors, similarly the skin differs in every individual depending on the dermal and epidermal histology and physiology. Histology means microscopic structure, such as fat, glands, etc. For example, depending on whether skin glands produce more or less secretions we end up having different levels of oily or dry skin. Perhaps some skin has more keratin on the surface, with more moisture, more elasticity, smaller pores; the result is a stronger barrier.

Physiology refers to the details of how the organs function, and remember the skin is the largest organ system in the body. Functions such as production of sweat, combat of infection, healing process and regulation of temperature are all considered skin physiological activities.

The ideal situation for any living organism is to be harmonious with every other living structure in the vicinity. The skin is one organ system in relation with many others in the body, like the circulatory or lymphatic systems. In turn the skin (medically known as the integumentary system) is in direct relationship with the external elements, like the sun and wind. The balance and end result of these relationships will have a cumulative effect on the appearance and viability of the skin.

Let's try to dissect this last statement. First it is important to grasp that all of the organ systems of the body, some way or another, have a direct relationship with the skin. For example; the circulatory system is the heart and all blood vessels. The termination of all vessels is the capillary, the very smallest tributary of this network. The capillary is found in the dermis. A problem with the circulatory system will be reflected in the appearance of the skin. Too much blood with wide open vessels will cause a flushing or red appearance. A sharp decrease in blood flow will cause a pale or bland appearance of the skin. The same goes for the nervous system. Continuous nervous stimulation can alter the appearance of the skin. Drastic changes like loss of hair, itchiness, skin breakouts, and acne can be directly proportional to excessive nervous expression.

It is important at this point to note that another role of the skin is to function as an interactive semipermeable structure to both secrete byproducts of internal metabolism (like sweat and oil), as well as shield us from the external elements... like the sun and the wind. How your skin performs these functions determines the outer appearance and skin type. For example, if there is insufficient production of natural skin oil, combined with over exposure to the wind or sun; the result is dry and scaly skin. The long term effect of this same scenario over an extended period leads to early and more pronounced signs of aging.

When there is an imbalance between the nutrients (for example Vitamin C, Vitamin E) and lubricants (natural oils) produced by the dermis, and the utilization and concentrations of these products in the epidermis, the result manifests itself in an altered skin appearance. Altered skin means unhealthy manifestations like, dry, scaly skin; or perhaps acne or rosacea. On the other hand a structure with perfect microscopic feature's such as pores of perfect dimensions, or natural oil in adequate concentrations will manifest as healthy glowing skin. In the perfect world your genetic make-up and habits are optimized to extend the shiny and glowing nature of our outer appearance for many years. The perfect skin is shiny, has an even pigment in whatever shade and has a tight appearance. This means that the production of oil is just right, never too shiny and never too dry. When you are exposed to the sun for a short period your skin tans evenly and does not burn easily. Also the perfect skin is tight and flexible with very few apparent wrinkles for any particular age. Imagine Sofia Loren or Halle Berry, they both have glowing shiny evenly pigmented skin free of wrinkles. Just as a good team is made up of members with different skills that share a common goal, the ideal skin has a moist strong outer surface combined with a formidable amount of supporting structures underneath.

The glistening appearance of the outer skin surface is a direct result of how the structures of the skin work together to give sustenance and support. Healthy and viable epithelium occurs because the organelles or microscopic organs like sweat glands, in the dermis produce the appropriate oils and lubricants. Concurrently the micro skeletal support system composed of fibrin protein elements in the dermis give a definitive structural semblance. One of the keys to ascertain skin types is the tensile strength, and this is determined by the structure in the dermis. We explained before how the fibrous elements are like tent poles of a tent. If they are not strong and bound the external surface will creep in and form a crease or wrinkle. The tensile strength of your skin is one of the elements we will categorize to determine your skin type.

The Skin Type Quiz

Step 1.

Can you identify with a specific lineage, heritage or ancestral origin?

Answer yes or no.
If the answer is yes continue with the following questions.

1.1 Are your descendants from the: (5 points)

- Mediterranean?
- Middle East?
- Caribbean?
- Polynesian?
- Central or South America?

1.2 Is your family of Native American, Oriental, or Indonesian decent? (4 points)

1.3 Do you consider yourself Caucasian, White or of European decent? (2 points)

1.4 Are you of African descent? (3 points)

1.5 Do you have blonde hair? (3 points)

1.6 Do you have hazel, blue or green eyes? (3 points)

1.7 Would you say you are of mixed heritage with a dark complexion? (4 points)

Beautiful skin is everyone's desire, and obtainable with varying degrees of effort depending on your genetic and physiologic characteristics.

Race or ethnicity is important, because as any Darwinian will explain, the body has adapted to geography and molded by intermingling of species. But more important is your own behavior, habits and interaction with the elements. We are all born with a given set of variables, (such as color, bone structure, melanin

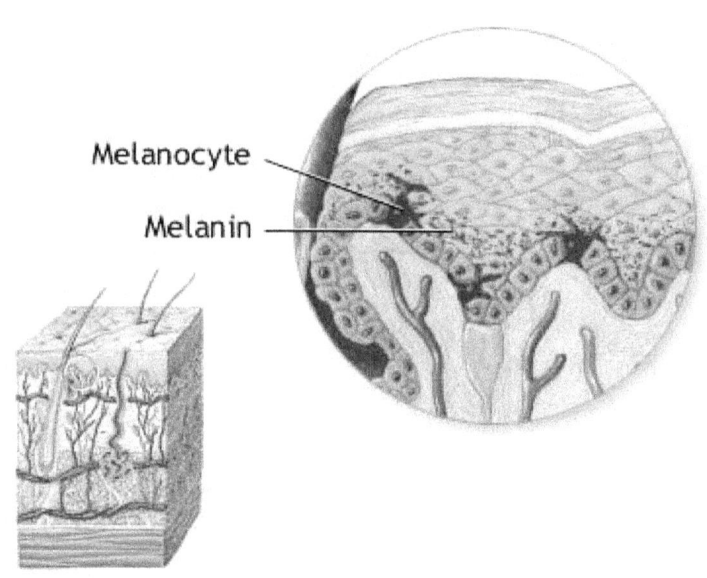

Melanocyte

Melanin

concentration) which do not necessarily determine a definitive skin appearance.

The color of your skin has very little to do with the type of skin you have, but it is important to understand how pigment is produced and what determines skin color. Each skin color reflects light and absorbs oils differently; therefore we should grasp the difference.

The color of your skin is determined by the amount of melanin, or pigment found in the deepest layer of the epithelium. A cell called the melanocyte produces and houses a dark secretion that gathers within the cell. This is the pigment that determines the color of your skin. For example, if melanin is produced in large quantities in an orderly fashion by a greater number of melanocytes, you are most likely of African descent. But, if there is a haphazard production in disorderly fashion, then this is a melanoma – a very malignant and aggressive lesion found both in fair and dark skinned people. You see, the same substance, produced by the same cell can either be a definition of race, or an abnormal manifestation, a disease state.

In the photo below observe the complex biochemical equations involved in the synthesis of melanin. This is not important for you to understand, only to illustrate how the deep understanding of a biologic process, like the production of pigment; can lead towards a logical approach in treating un-wanted pigment, acne, wrinkles or rash.

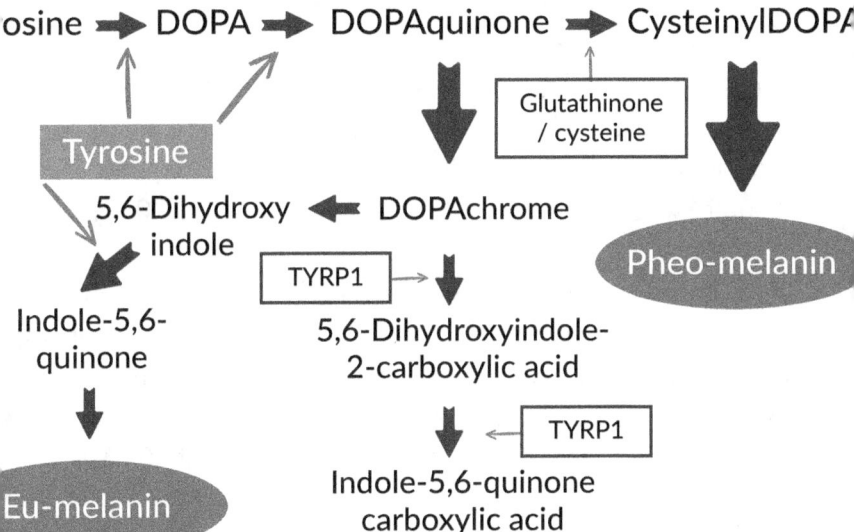

The reason for looking back, then around is to grasp the concept of genetic influence. Who we are, and what kind of skin we have, is very much influenced by our genetic structure.

Step2.

Is your skin sensitive or resistant?

2.1 Have you ever had an allergic skin reaction, causing itchiness, bumps or blisters? Yes or No. If no give yourself. (5 points)

2.2 Did you have acne? If No, give yourself 5 points. If only during teen years and scant, 4 points. If acne outbreaks were moderate and extended into the twenties, 3 points. If moderate and still occasionally have adult breakouts, 2 points. If severe with residual scaring in adulthood, but no further adult episodes, 1 point. Finally if severe with scaring and occasional adult breakouts. (0 points)

2.3 Have you ever had a diagnosed skin disease like psoriasis, lupus, rashes, hives, nevi, pigmented bumps, actinic keratosis, basal cell carcinoma, squamous cell carcinoma or melanoma? If no, give yourself 5 points. For any answer take 1 point away from 5, and if you have 5 or more of the above give yourself. (0 points)

Any race has tendencies to either develop acne or not. Pigmented lesions (such as birthmarks and freckles) can be seen in all creeds and colors. Therefore the first lesson in skin typing is looking beyond the color and focus on physical findings in any color's.

Step3.

You and your surroundings. Once you have an insight into what you are made of, take another look around you. Where are you? In a dry or humid place, Miami or Las Vegas? How do you feel in your surrounding? Do you sweat profusely?

Is your skin dry, or sunburned? Your surroundings can offer hints as to your skin type, by the way your skin reacts to the external environment.

So please answer the following questions

3.1 Do you live in a dry or humid location? Please categorize your usual surroundings. Tropical, Desert, Seasonal, predominantly winter, predominantly summer. Once you categorize your surrounding please answer the following.

3.2 Do you live in the same like location as you were born in?
   -If yes give yourself. (5 points)

3.3 How many times have you had sunburn severe enough to cause discomfort, blistering and pealing?

   - Never, (5 points)
   - Less than 5 times, (4 points)
   - Less than 10 times, (3 points)
   - Every summer on one occasion (2 points)
   - Often even though using sun screens (1 point)
   - Too many to remember, hardly ever used sun screen during youth, (0 points)

3.4 Have you ever been exposed to cold wind and breeze with formation of skin burns and blisters?

- If no, give yourself (5 points)

Well we're almost finished, just a few more questions.

Step4.
Is your skin oily or dry?
Everyone's skin is one of these.

Both extremes you will give yourself 0.

The middle ground (combination skin) in this case will render the highest score of 5.

The natural oils produced by the glands in the dermis are the single most important source of natural protection, nutrition and hydration. Balance is everything in this case. An over production will open one up towards propensity of clogging pores and development of acne and later rosacea. The perfect balance makes for a shiny healthy glow devoid of lumps, bumps and pigments.

The very last step involves a simple evaluation and question.

Step5.
How old were you when you noticed your first wrinkle?

If your answer is 42 or above give yourself a 5.

- 39 and above 4.
- 35 and above 3.
- 32 and above 2.
- 29 and above 1.

- 27 and below 0.

Tally the score

We will divide the skin types into four categories depending on your skin quiz score.

In the next chapter we will discuss the skin products and regimens which will suit each category.

Class I, Wonder skin. "If your score is 37 or above you are in a unique and optimal category. Chances are no matter what you do, you're one step ahead of everyone else. This group has a glowing healthy appearance skin, and naturally looks younger than their age.

Class II, "Easy fix" category. If your score is 22 or above, you look better than most, but more important is that with a little care and attention drastic improvements are readily accessible. This group is characterized by a natural tendency to look good with minimal effort. Imagine a bit of support with the appropriate products and daily regimen, surpassing the 'wonder skin group' is definitely possible.

Class III, 'Watch yourself and pamper yourself'. If your score is 14 or above, than this is a less than optimal category. It doesn't mean that there is no solution, there definitely is; but you will have to work hard to achieve an optimal effect. In these class constant preventative remedies, daily applications of different products as well as exfoliations, and possible more invasive strategies will be warranted eventually.

Class IV, 'Road Warrior'. If you scored below 13 points than buckle your seat belt and hold on. Only with aggressive and constant attention to the several issues present in the skin will modify the accrued damage. This group wills most likely benefit most with more invasive strategies.

We will discuss in detail how to approach a personal skin remedy plan to look younger and feel better about yourself. The only thing that has no solution is death, so we will work with you no matter the skin quiz score.

This book is about helping you look young... into your middle age and beyond. You can be absolutely sure that if you live long enough the dreaded wrinkle will make a personal appearance on your face. To actually make a plan, a game plan, first take score. Get to know yourself by peeling away the outer structure and glancing within.

The skin is always just epidermis, dermis and subcutaneous tissue.

Our genes and how we react to our surroundings make up the intrinsic and extrinsic factors that determine the different skin types. The basic approach to establishing a skin type is to judge how durable and tough the outer shield is, and how much substance is produced by the glandular factory underlying the surface within the dermis. Simply spoken, how tough, how moist your skin is varying degrees of strength and humidity, the end result is your specific skin type.

Now consider your relationship with the sun. Not in the way the Egyptian pharos meant, but the way a surfer on the beach looks at it. Take note of how much time you spend with direct and prolonged exposure to the sun. Reflect on how often you have gone sun bathing throughout your life, without using sun blocks or moisturizers afterwards.

Skin type is very much determined by how we react, tolerate and expose ourselves to the sun. Sunburn, heat blisters, tanning are all reactions to the ultraviolet rays of the sun. Later on we will quantify our reflection by answering a few questions.

In my research the work of Dr. Leslie Bauman was very enlightening. Not only does she reside in my favorite city of Miami, but also her credentials are impeccable. She offers some insight into how to determine what type of skin you have which can be found in her book "The Skin Type Solution".

I have my own approach to determine skin type by considering the physiopathology (abnormal results) of skin reactions and how there is distinct variance and common bonds between all of them.

The inflammatory cells present in the skin can alter and determine the specific gross and microscopic appearance for each skin type. One known scientific truth is that behind all reactive skin lesions is a state of inflammation. Inflamed means irritated, red, and itchy. Perhaps it manifests as a bump, red spot or pimple. In any event if you look with a microscope you will see different kinds of white blood cells, or inflammatory cells where they do not belong. Different types and amounts of inflammatory and how many of them, and where they are found in the skin will manifest into a very benign and simple problem with an easy solution; or perhaps a chronic and predisposed situation requiring extensive professional help. We do not pretend to cover all diseases of the skin and the appropriate treatment, but there is hope that the common and solvable problems can be dealt with in a structured and logical fashion

The treatment and prevention of wrinkles, dry skin, rashes, sun exposure will be determined on an individual basis. Before you can empirically suggest any cream, vitamin or invasive process to heal the skin, you are obligated to establish your skin type.

Skin Types	Characterisitcs	Genetic Origin
1	never tans, always burns easily, skin particularly light, freckles, redish hair (all babies and children)	Scandinavian, Celtic
2	skin somehow darker than Type1, freckles rare, tans slightly, high inclination to sunburn	Caucasians
3	skin light / light brown, no freckles, good tanning ability, very low inclination to sunburn	Central Europe
4	skin light-brown to olive, no freckles, very good tanning ability, very low inclination to sunburn	South Mediteranean, South American
5	skin olive in color, sun insensitive skin, very low inclination to sunburn	Middle Eastern, Asia, some Hispanics and Afro-American
6	skin deeply pigmented, sun insensitive skin, never burns	African, Afro-American

To just consider the ethnic typing of skin, is not accurate enough for our tastes. This will suffice for the first portion of your exercise in looking at the genetic makeup of you.

Take some time to digest what we have covered until now, and get ready to answer some simple questions honestly.

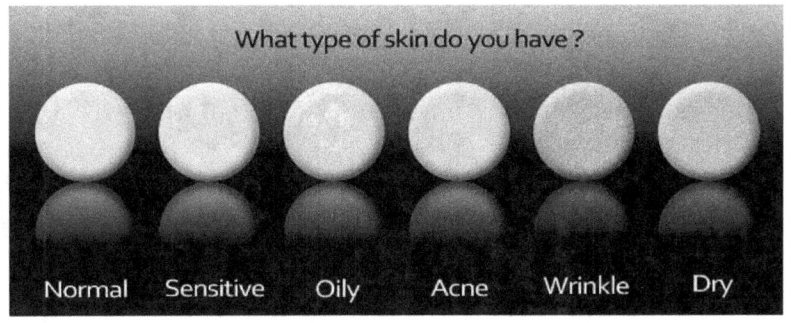

In this photo observe that the point is not to determine the outer appearance, but to establish a general characteristic based on past and present tendencies.

These very categories can be found in a person of any color.

These photos demonstrate the entire rainbow of colors, but each can be dry, oily, wrinkled, or with acne. You should have some idea of the characteristics which will determine your skin type.

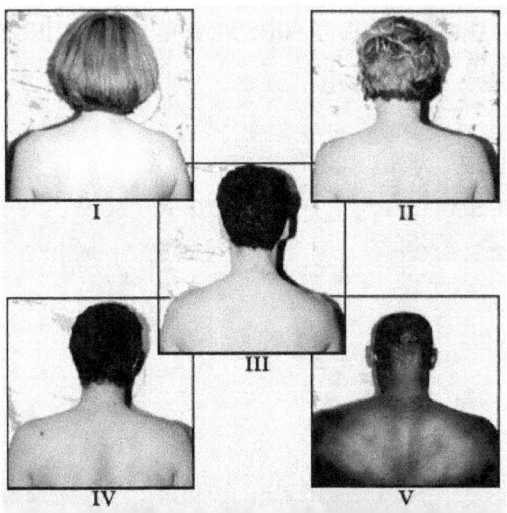

Think of your past and reactions to food, sun, creams and jewelry the purpose of this entire exercise is to pick and choose the personal approach to take care of only your skin.

The first thing I usually ask a patient is, "are you allergic to anything?"

Meanwhile there must be focused effort to evaluate the what, how, when and where any symptom or sign began

Basically you have a few simple decisions to make based on all the information we have gathered together.

1. How tough is your shield?

2. How tight is the skin that binds you?

3. Is your skin moist most of the time?

How much time do you spend with direct exposure to the sun.

4. How often have you searched for an antihistamine, anti-itch cream or acne medication?

5. In photographs, does your skin have a shiny appearance?

Let's tally up your score.

- If your score is _____than see schedule A.

- If your score is_____than se schedule B.

Chapter Fourteen
Solve the Problem

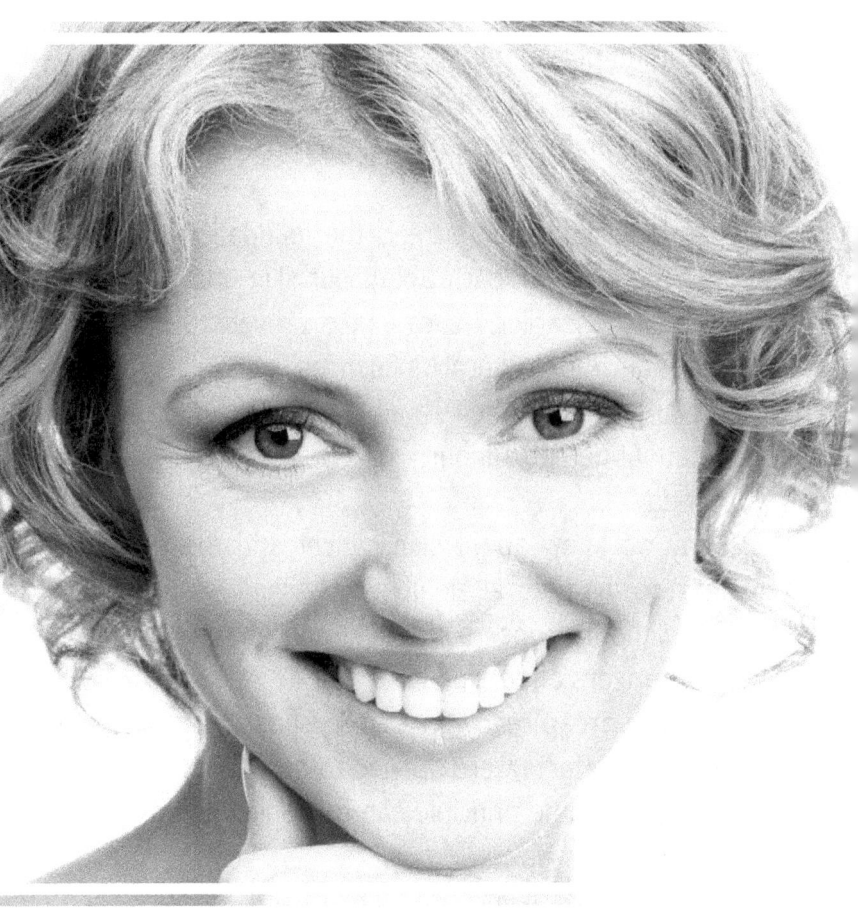

Solutions and Treatment Plans

No matter what skin type you are, or what genetic constitution; we all need to follow certain basic principles to maintain and achieve optimum skin appearance.

Like everything else in life, some of us have to work harder than others. The differences are quantitative and not qualitative. That is to say, we should all follow the same basic recommendations, and seek professional help when there is no improvement.

In the chapters preceding we wrote about the environment and how the sun, wind and varying exposures to each affect our appearance.

Therefore, common sense is the foundation of this plan. The earlier in life we learn about our skin and how and why it changes, the earlier we can take preventative measures. Generational and cultural influences seem to mold our behavioral patterns. When I was a teenager, no one seemed to care about getting sunburn, beyond the pain it would cause the next day.

Today we know about skin cancer and the gradients of exposure to the natural elements. My children never went in the sun without proper sun block, and always were treated with moisturizers after exposure.

So, they are already in better shape, simply because practical known facts were applied to daily living.

Exactly the same principle can be applied to your diet and choices along the way.

The scientific facts are there, you simply need to incorporate them into your life.

One thing is certain; the skin is the largest organ system in the human body. The skin is part and parcel, intimately connected with every organ system.

To separate the heart, lungs, stomach, brain, etc... from the functions of the skin is useful to understand independent physiology. What is the point? Well, the issue is that your diet, exercise, nervous conditions are all reflected in the skin.

The components of a healthy life style are not up for debate. We all know what they are.

So, before we even talk about topical applications, we should be clear that there is more to skin care than a cream or two.

*Step One can be referred to a sensible life style, with the proper diet, exercise, outlook and preventative measures to lay down the foundation for healthy skin.

*Step two is a proper cleansing of the skin twice daily. There are scores of cleansing agents on the shelves of stores on every corner.

Our focus is to educate the reader in choosing the right one. An effective cleanser must be formulated to remove dirt, oil, environmental pollutants and any residues from makeup.

All skin types, except the highly sensitive, respond to a 'Glycolic Cleanser', in other words, one which contains glycolic acid.

The educated consumer will take a close look at the ingredients to make sure that there are other essential components in the products you choose.

We strongly recommend the addition of soothing anti-aging natural green tea, along with Aloe, Alpha Hydroxyl acids and any other anti-oxidants with a proven track record.

Please note that we have discussed these in the Love potion #9 chapters.

The application technique is just as relevant as the cleanser of choice. Try to use your finger tips to apply with a gentle circular motion.

After a few minutes, rinse with room temperature water and pat dry with a clean cloth.

*Step three is an extended rinse after the cleansing of the exfoliated process. By the way, do you know what exfoliates means? Well it's a fancy way of saying deep cleansing.

Literally it means to debride dead cells and waist. Remember that the skin is composed of layers of different cells.

The cells are constantly going through a cycle of birth and death, a microscopic reincarnation.

After the deep cleansing the remaining superficial surface is extra sensitive and vulnerable.

At the same time the skin is now ready for a balancing regimen to bring the pH. levels back to normal.

It's up to you to pick the right product. Try to discern through the ingredients, and go to the 'Toner' section of the skin care department.

We strongly recommend a 3% glycolic toner. The key ingredients to look for are Aloe, Glycolic Acid, Cucumber, and Witch Hazel. Keep it as simple as possible.

The whole purpose of this phase of treatment is to promote continuous cell turnover which in turn will promote rejuvenation.

The skin type of each individual will determine the variant treatments and toners applied.

If your skin has an uneven appearance, or areas that

appear darker or dryer than other areas; you will need additional treatment. One such example is the use of Alpha Arbutin Serum.

This compound tends to mimic hydroquinone. This serum contains high concentrations of all natural ingredients; such as Bearberry, Kojic,Licorice ans Seaweed extract.

Age and additional complications such as acne, rosacea or excessive oily appearance; will in turn require additional care.

If you have had or have the tendency towards acne, than it is important to add an Alpha Beta Toner after a deep cleaning.

The key ingredients to look for are Salicylic Acid, Lactic Acid, Ginseng and Butylcarbamate.

In the event that you have sun damaged skin, which is highly sensitive; a Green Tea Toner will do the trick.

Now look for a product with Green Tea Extract, Glycerin Hydantoin. This is best used as a spray that can be used several times throughout the day, just to freshen up a bit. The skin will feel refreshed and calm after each application.

If you are over 40 years old, and have already started, seeing the appearance of deeper wrinkles, then an anti-aging Moisturizer is called for. This book is all about simplicity, it's not meant for a detailed medical plan. That being said, we recommend any cream which contains Octioxate, and Titanium Dioxide. Other ingredients will make the cream more skin type specific. Vitamin A, Alpha Lipoic Acid,Shea Butter; and all of the other contents mentioned in the 'love potion #9' chapter will add to the positive outcomes.

After careful review of all scientific and cosmetic literature relevant to our research; we think that a personal consultation can be of great value. So with the purchase of this book we offer a one-time free consultation, specific for you.

By using submitting the questionnaire in the skin type chapter, and a skype interview, we will be able to assist you further.

Conclusions
"Live a peaceful and harmonious existence"

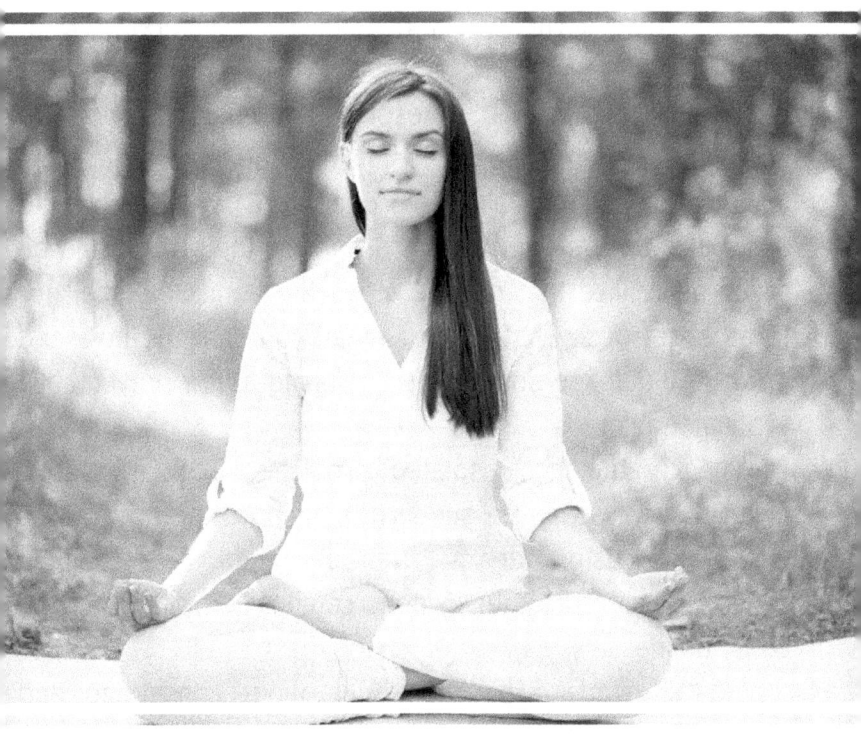

So Now What ?

After reading all previous chapters you should now have some fundamental knowledge of the basic structure and function of skin. The skin is a perfectly designed barrier and reflects our constitution and life style: composed of an ever changing variable cell structure, constantly reacting to the envoirment, and versatile enough to respond to care or abuse.

This book is meant to be didactic, a conversation with each reader, with the expectation that a self-analysis is ongoing from chapter one. So, do you have an idea of your skin type? No need to be dermatologist or scientist to understand your own skin.

Take advantage of the resources given in this book to figure out your own past, present and future, of your skin. Immediately begin to take the proper steps to decelerate the aging process. You must put your feet on the ground and be practical, realize that no one stops the hands of time, nor takes a get over. That doesn't mean you can't be bold and attack the damage done, while beginning a new preventative protection plan.

The treatment of isolated problems like dark spots, acne, rosacea, pimples, sunburn, sagging skin and wrinkles should be custom designed as per need. The common ground is altered by the genetic composition, life style and consciousness.

We all need to be thoughtful about conserving and protecting our skin. Like everything else in life, some will have to work harder at it than others. Many have natural protection and strong constitution, they need a minimum effort. Some have severe damage due to a life time of abuse, and predisposed weakness to rapid reactive and deteriorating changes.

Our skin is a semi permeable armor, which interacts and simultaneously protects us from nature. Taking into considerations all variants of skin types and life styles, and the need to tailor each plan, let us take a look at the basic common approaches to treatment of skin problems.

That person, who is so fortunate to have a lightly pigmented tight skin with no history of acne or freckles, can completely relax. Then there is the other end of the spectrum, dry or oily skin, loose , history of acne and multiple sun burns; you guys have to be on your toes, aggressive and relentless.

There are common variable.

Cleanliness and cleansing with the right cleansing products, is at the top of the list.

Take time to learn and identify the ingredients you should look for, and those to avoid.

A cleanser should contain aloe vera, benzoyl peroxide, some retinol, antioxidants, and more...but should never have acetone, or alcohol.

Those with very dry skin should look for a cooling cucumber base and some sort of cold cream to use for cleansing.

You can add a weekly mask to your routine, and there are many to choose from, we recommend sulfur containing product or one which is a soothing gel base.

Sun protection is key. A daily moisturizer with SPF 15, eucerin, aloe vera, salyxilic acid, and ginger is ideal; again the type of sun block will be dictated by the akin type.

Moisturizers are very important in reestablishing and maintaining a healthy skin glow.

There are a score of moisturizing lotions that are suitable. Many of the anti-wrinkle creams on the market which enhance natural moisture, and generate our own reactive process must be looked at on an individual basis.

Stay away from any product with obvious false claims to make you look instantly younger. This is not going to happen, there are no snake vendor magic formulas on the market, that really work.

However, caffeine, Vitamin E, ginseng, lactic acid and Coenzyme Q, can all be helpful.

Those with damages skin, very dry and a long history of issues need to vary the day from the night moisturizing regimens. Cocoa butter, Canola oil, high aloe vera content, olive oil and Shea butter are strongly recommended.

Add on to this regimen serums masks, infiltration, as needed. The whole purpose of this aggressive skin care is to keep out irritants and the natural barrier strength.

Avoiding inflammation or the infiltration of lymphocytes into the dermis is key to your success.

The task at hand is diurnal, twice a day. A morning and night time regimen.

A perpetual routine of cleansing, skin cream applications, sun screens, and moisturizers.

Please note that for damaged skin we strongly recommend physician supervised treatments like chemical peels, microdermabrasion and prescription strength products.

Meanwhile you must focus on the goal, which is the restoration and enhancement of the natural protective skin barrier.

There is a light at the end of the tunnel, and it's not a freight train coming toward you.

Since the skin is changing daily, there is actual birth and death of cells every day; therefore with proper protection from irritants and damage, a whole new barrier can be generated over time.

From the bottom portion of the most superficial skin segment, the epidermis, new cells are born every day.

These cells slowly migrate towards the surface, replacing the older cells,

These older squamous cells loose their ability to reproduce and slough off as a keratin mass devoid of nucleus or DNA. So, the point is, by implementing a twice a day routine tailored to specific needs, according to skin type, and skin status, you can achieve a fresh new look.

Now let's be very clear, there is more to this than cleansers and creams.

Each reader has to change his daily habits. There are many choices to be made. Like anything, the more you give the more you get, and so instant karma is applied to skin care.

For the optimum effect, and life changing results, yes you must actually eliminate a lot of bad habits and replace those hinderances with positivity.

So you get what you give, no one is absolved cheaply from the sins of the past.

How badly do you want to slow down the aging process?

How much do you want to look and feel younger and healthier?

If yes, yes, younger, healthier, happier... are your answers, then here are my fanatical suggestions.

You are what you eat. You are what you drink.

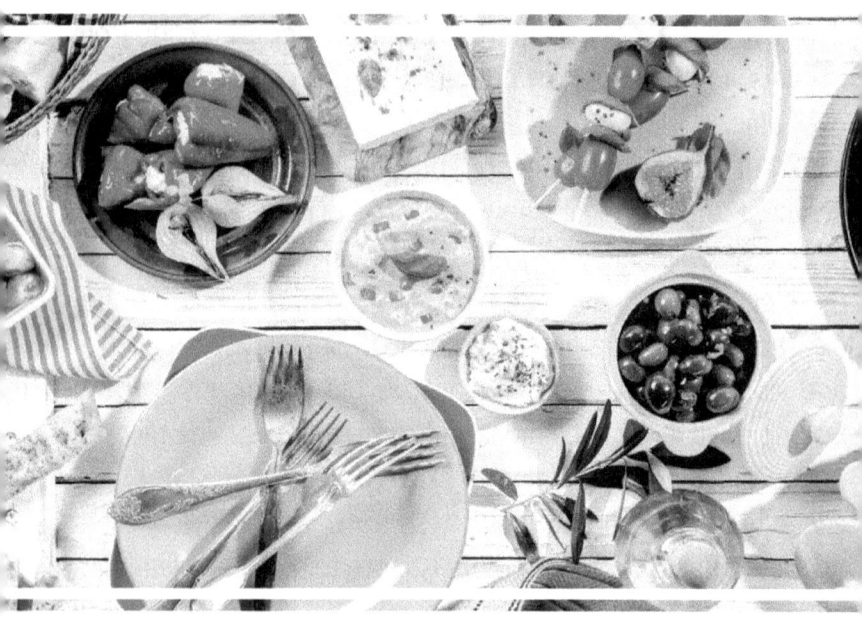

If you become a vegetarian, stop consuming all intoxicants, and dedicate time each day to meditation, your life will change.

Live a peaceful and harmonious existence with all living beings, you will see tremendous changes, including healthier skin.

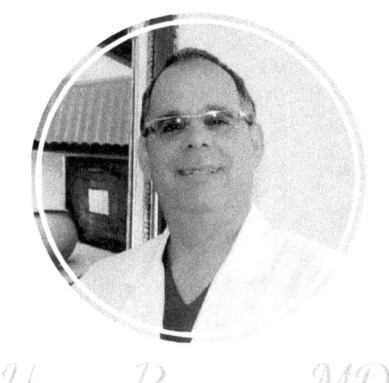

Hugo Romeu, MD

● Chant and be happy ●

Hare Krishna Hare Krishna
Krishna Krishna Hare Hare
Hare Rama Hare Rama
Rama Rama Hare Hare

Dr.hugoromeu@yahoo.com
www.RCEGroupUSA.com
www.romeuclinical.com
www.pharmrce.com.mx
www.farmaciarce.com
www.theclinical.org
www.rerelab.com
www.reliableresearchlaboratory.com

Beauty & Skin
Reflexions in health care

NOTES

About the author

Dr. Hugo Romeu received formal training in experimental laboratory medicine at several prestigious institutions such as Roswell Park Memorial Institute, State University of New York and Cook County Hospital. He has published written protocols and participated in study designs in all phases of research, from pre-clinical animal trials to late phase studies. Over the last 32 years he has completed 672 trials, the majority phase one and bioequivalence.

His clients include the largest pharmaceutical companies as well as local smaller members in the arena.

Dr. Romeu is currently the managing partner and is on board around the clock to make sure that Reliable Research Lab maintains the high expectations this industry demands.